MUSCLES, MOBILITY &

MASTER MUSCLE ANATOMY, MUSCL MOBILITY, AND MUSCULAR STREI

ISBN: 9798455812705

Published by www.strengthandconditioningcourse.com

Copyright © 2020 Strength and Course Limted

The moral right of this author has been asserted.

All rights reserved. No part of this publication may be reproduced, distributed, or transmitted in any form or by any means, including photocopying, recording, or other electronic or mechanical methods, without the prior written permission of the publisher, except in the case of brief quotations embodied in critical reviews and certain other non-commercial uses permitted by copyright law.

www.strengthandconditioningcourse.com

Facebook & Instagram: @strengthandconditioningcourse

Cover Image Copyright: Shutterstock: SciePro & Jacob Lund

Image Copyright: Strength and Conditioning Course

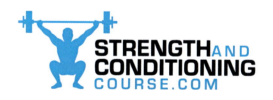

CONTENTS

TABLE OF CONTENTS

4

INTRODUCTION

The fitness industry has traditionally been dominated by weight loss and body transformations. As a whole, this is not a bad thing because body composition is fundamental to physical health and wellbeing. However, I often feel that far too much emphasis is put on aesthetics (the way we look), and not enough focus is placed on overall musculoskeletal health, i.e., the health of our muscles, tendons, ligaments, and skeleton.

Of course, body composition goals are brilliant motivators and will likely be the most popular goals within the fitness industry for a long-time to come. However, if people placed a little more emphasis on long-term musculoskeletal health, it would result in better training (and diet), more consistency, and ultimately a healthier and happier population.

We all get dealt a genetic hand, and we have to play that hand the best we can. Unfortunately, some hands are better than others, and some games are far tougher than others. You may be more predisposed to specific injuries and ailments, or you may sustain injuries that have lifelong impacts. Life is NOT fair, and hurdles will be thrown in your way. However, each and every one of us is given ONE body, and it is our responsibility to look after our body and its long-term health.

How do we look after our long-term health?

It is pretty simple. Eat a well-balanced diet that consists of a wide variety of nutritious foods, don't do things to an unhealthy excess, and MOVE – doing all this won't guarantee a long life, but you will be playing your hand well and maximizing the years you do have.

In this book, we are not going to concern ourselves with nutrition. However, we are going to talk about movement in incredible detail.

Socrates said, "No man has the right to be an amateur in the matter of physical training. It is a shame for a man to grow old without seeing the beauty and strength of which his body is capable" – this applies to both men and women.

Of course, not everyone can be an expert, which is why we have professionals that specialize. However, you have a duty to YOUR body to understand how to keep your musculoskeletal system in good health. And yes, there is a fair bit to learn, but I am not an academic, and I don't write for academics. I was a physical training instructor in the British infantry, and I have run a gym ever since. I write for people that are willing to learn, and I stand by Albert Einstein's quote, "If you can't explain it simply, you don't understand it well enough." So, yes, this book deals with complex terminology and training principles and will be helpful to both elite-level coaches and athletes. However, it is also written with the layman in mind.

This book looks at the muscles that facilitate specific movements and takes an in-depth look at how these muscles impact joint function and movement as a whole.

We will start by looking at mobility and flexibility. From there, we will first look at what corrective exercise is. We will then define the fundamental human movements and begin with brace and posture.

MUSCLE TERMINOLOGY

- **Origin:** The origin is attached to a fixed bone that usually doesn't move during contraction. It is often described as the proximal attachment, meaning it is closer to the centre or midline of the body – muscles may have more than one origin, for example, the triceps have 3, and the biceps have 2.

- **Insertion:** The insertion is the attachment to a bone that usually moves during contraction. It is often described as the distal attachment, meaning further from the centre or midline of the body.

- **Prime Movers / Agonists:** These are the primary muscles that perform the desired action. For example, the biceps during a biceps curl.

- **Antagonists:** These are the muscles that oppose the agonist, for example, the triceps during a biceps curl.

- **Synergists:** These are the muscles that assist the agonist, for example, the brachioradialis.

- **Fixators:** These are the muscles that stabilize the body during the movement, for example, the deltoid during a biceps curl.

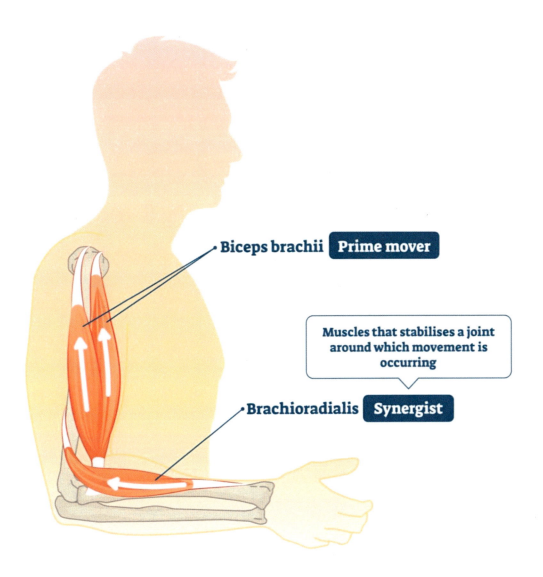

Biceps brachii — **Prime mover**

Muscles that stabilises a joint around which movement is occurring

Brachioradialis — **Synergist**

If we can visualize the muscles and understand which joints the muscle(s) cross, we can understand their function. And this is why I designed our unique muscle manual in the way I did.

You also get Version 2 of our Muscle Manual, which lists the muscles:

- Origin.

- Insertion.

- Action.

- Antagonist.

- Innervation.

- Blood Supply.

- Daily Use.

- Gym Use.

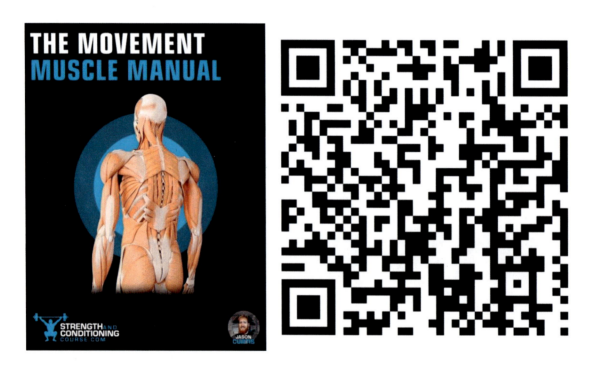

https://courses.strengthandconditioningcourse.com/p/muscle-manual-pdf

Check out the link below to grab a paperback copy of The Movement Muscle Manual:

mybook.to/musclemanual

Once we know what the muscle does, we can look at what day-to-day activities, training methods, and sporting actions work it. We can look at what muscles assist and stabilize the action and what muscles oppose it.

But why is it pertinent to understand which muscles assist, stabilize and oppose each other?

- If a muscle is tense or prone to injury, it could be overworking and, therefore, building strength in the muscles that assist the action could be well received.

- If a muscle is potentially being overused, it can also impact the opposing muscle(s). Therefore, programming more work on the opposing muscle group can have great benefits. For example, we often program more hamstring work for athletes with tense, overworked quadriceps.

- If a movement is unstable, we could spend more time working the muscles that fixate the action.

This all being said, we want to increase the load tolerance of all our muscles. The more strength (load tolerance) a muscle has, the more stress it can accommodate – if a muscle lacks the strength to accommodate the stress, it may become tense.

The way we maximize musculoskeletal health is with the progressive development of strength in our structures. This is best done with a wide variety of bodyweight and resistance exercises. We also compound this with a wide variety of mobility and flexibility techniques.

In this small section, the term "tense" has been used a lot. However, this term is subjective, and often, words like this get thrown around with little thought of the deeper cause. Therefore, we will break this down in the section Mobility & Flexibility.

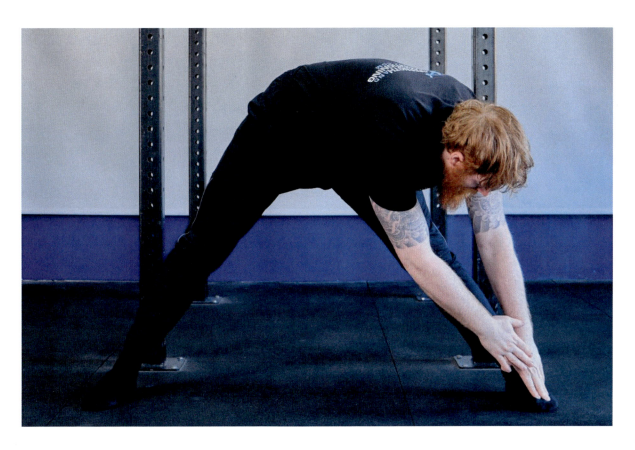

HUMAN MOVEMENT & THE PREREQUISITE

THE BIG 8

There are seven basic human movements and one precursor – The BIG 8:

1. **Brace:** The ability to create tension and maintain a position. Bracing is vital in maintaining posture, both statically (stood still) and dynamically (moving).

2. **Hinge:** Bending at the hips while keeping the knees straight and maintaining a neutral spine (unbent and untwisted).

3. **Squat:** Bending at the hips, knees, and ankles while maintaining a neutral spine.

4. **Lunge:** Single-leg exercises that work the legs independently from one another (unilateral).

5. **Push:** Pushing with the upper body.

6. **Pull:** Pulling with the upper body. The deadlift exercise is often classified as a "Pull" exercise (pulling from the floor). However, the deadlift can be better classified as a hinge exercise as the emphasis is on hip extension.

7. **Rotate**: Rotation is primarily performed at the hips and shoulders (ball and socket joints) and at the spine through a series of facet joints. These structures can work in isolation or together to produce a greater range of motion (ROM).

8. **Gait:** Walking, running, and carries (locomotion).

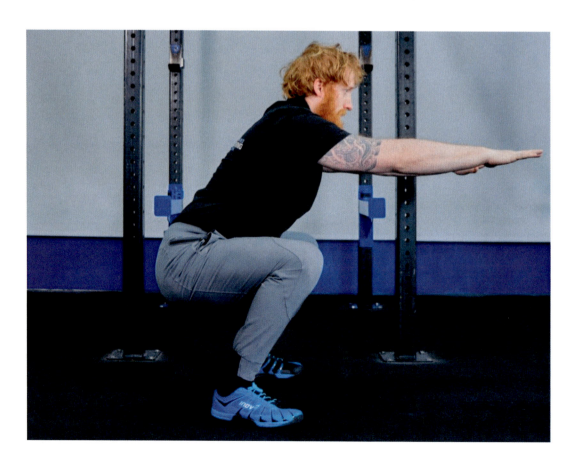

We develop all the above movements with compound exercises, which work multiple joints and muscle groups, and isolation exercises that work single joint actions and target the individual muscles responsible for performing the actions.

The ideal way to order the exercises is to start with primary lifts, move on to assistance lifts, and finish with auxiliary lifts.

- **Primary Lifts/Exercises** are compound exercises. They are of utmost importance in terms of exercise selection as they usually work through the greatest ROM with the heaviest loads and, therefore, require the most effort, i.e., barbell back squats, deadlifts, or press variations.

- **Assistance Lifts/Exercises** are often referred to as accessory exercises and are also compound movements. They are chosen to develop specific movements or muscle groups that help you to perform the primary lift or specific sporting actions.

- **Auxiliary Lifts/Exercises** are single-joint (isolation) exercises. They are chosen to help develop your ability to perform the primary lift or specific sporting actions.

These exercises usually involve isotonic contractions, meaning the muscles are shortening and lengthening as we progress through the range of motion.

- **Concentric Contraction:** Where the muscle shortens.

- **Eccentric Contraction:** Where the muscle lengthens.

We can also perform these exercises isometrically, where we hold the position and there is no change in muscle length. Examples include planks, wall sits, or simply pausing during any movement – these exercises can be described as "brace" exercises.

Note: The eccentric phase is much stronger than the concentric phase – you might be able to lower a weight with control during a squat but are unable to come back up.

The eccentric phase is also responsible for most of the delayed onset muscle soreness (DOMS) we experience days after training.

DOMS:

- Pain/discomfort and stiffness felt in the muscles several hours or days after exercise - the soreness is felt most strongly 24-72 hours after exercise.

- Eccentric contractions are known to cause greater DOMS.

- The key to preventing DOMS is progressive training and good training frequency – DOMS increase when there is a spike in volume/intensity or a sudden change in the type of stressors included in the session.

- DOMS should not be chased – muscle soreness is NOT an accurate indicator of a "good session."

Coming from a prolonged rest period to even moderate training is essentially a spike in stress, and it is not uncommon for an athlete to suffer with notable DOMS even after a short period of inactivity. However, DOMS can have a negative impact on the training plan and therefore, should be limited – build resilience progressively.

Here are tables that illustrate the different joint actions that the body is capable of:

Action	Description	Action	Description
Flexion	Bending a body part.	**Extension**	Straightening a body part
Abduction	Moving a body part away from the midline.	**Adduction**	Moving a body part towards the midline.
Rotation	Circular movement around a bone.	**Circumduction**	Cone-shaped movement.
Lateral Flexion	Bending to the side.	**Lateral Extension**	Returning straight from a side bend position.
Horizontal Flexion	Moving a body part horizontally towards the midline.	**Horizontal extension**	Moving a body part horizontally away from the midline.
Elevation	Upwards movement of a body part.	**Depression**	Downwards movement of a body part.
Protraction	Forwards movement of a body part.	**Retraction**	Backwards movement of a body part.
Plantarflexion	Pointing the toes downwards.	**Dorsiflexion**	Pointing the toes upwards.
Pronation	Rotation of the forearm so the palm faces downwards.	**Supination**	Rotation of the forearm so the palm faces upwards.
Inversion	Moving the sole of the foot to face inwards.	**Eversion**	Moving the sole of the foot to face outwards.

Notes:

- Rotation is split into two categories, internal (medial) and external (lateral) rotation.

- Horizontal flexion and extension are also referred to as horizontal adduction and abduction.

- Pronation and supination can also be used to describe the action at the ankle, i.e., Pronation = eversion and supination = inversion – when someone is described as "over-pronating", they usually show a flat arch with more weight placed onto the inner side of the ball of the foot.

Typical ranges of motion:

Joint Action	Degrees of Motion	Joint Action	Degrees of Motion
Shoulder:			
Flexion	160	Extension	50
Internal Rotation	45	External Rotation	90
Abduction	180		
Elbow:			
Flexion	160	Extension	0
Hip:			
Flexion	120	Extension	0-10
Abduction	40	Adduction	15
Internal Rotation	45	External Rotation	45
Knee:			
Flexion	140	Extension	0
Ankle:			
Plantarflexion	45	Dorsiflexion	20

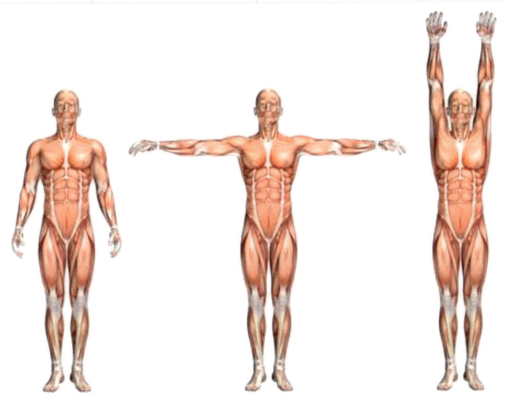

CORRECTIVE EXERCISE

Corrective exercise is a specialism where an in-depth knowledge of anatomy and biomechanics is used to prescribe specific exercises to fix movement limitations and compensations.

This book shows you how to teach fundamental movement patterns, correct faulty movement, and improve musculoskeletal health and performance.

It is NORMAL for there to be muscle imbalances and asymmetries (differences in strength and size between muscle groups and sides of the body). We should be cautious when it comes to labelling someone's movement as "dysfunctional" – some of the best athletes in the world have prominent imbalances. You don't want someone to leave a session feeling self-conscious and demotivated.

However, muscle imbalances, weaknesses, and mobility restrictions can result in compensation patterns, a higher risk of injury, and a reduction in performance. It is amazing how a slight change in positioning can greatly improve performance.

When we understand which muscles work together to perform a movement and which muscles oppose them, we better understand how to target them specifically, which helps us optimize performance, i.e., strength and hypertrophy (muscle building), and manage injuries.

Here are just a few of the key areas we will look at:

KEY AREAS		
• Anterior / Posterior / Lateral Pelvic Tilts.	• Ribcage Flare.	• Winged Scapula.
• Hyper-lordosis and Lower Cross Syndrome.	• Knee Valgus.	• Flaring Elbows During Horizontal Press.
• Hyper-Kyphosis and Upper Cross Syndrome.	• Pronation Distortion Syndrome.	• Overhead Immobility.
• Flat Back and Sway Back Posture.	• Hip Shifts.	• Overhead Instability.
• Over-Pronation and Supination of the Feet.	• The Good Morning Fault.	• Elevated Shoulders.
• Chest Breathing.	• Quad Dominance.	• Uneven Shoulders.
• Lack of Squat Depth.	• Anterior Knee Pain.	• Thoracic Rotation Immobility.
• Excessive Forward Lean During the Squat.	• Single-Leg Instability.	• Running Mechanics.
• The Butt Wink.	• Poor Hinge Mechanics.	• Foot Strike.
	• Lack of Lat Engagement During Deadlift.	

POSTURE

Static posture is the position someone holds their body in while standing, sitting, or lying, but is most commonly assessed in a standing position – dynamic posture refers to your positioning while performing movements.

For many years, some health and fitness professionals have promoted the utterly unrealistic notion that we should be in what is classed as "good posture" at all times, with our head and shoulders retracted (pulled back), chest proud (pushed out), and our spine neutral (unbent and untwisted). However, it is key to understand that it is fine to bend, twist and slouch. Ultimately the best posture is the next posture – spending hours in even the most ergonomic (efficiency and comfort) position is going to get sore and uncomfortable.

Although a draconian level of maintaining "good" posture is a little silly, there are clearly optimal positions for someone to take while static (standing in line) or performing an action (a deadlift) – optimal posture is often described as the "neutral" position where the least stress is placed on the joints and the surrounding structures.

No, having rounded shoulders or forward head posture is not a sure sign of a predisposition to injury, if only it were that simple. However, try taking your arms overhead while your upper back and shoulders are rounded (protracted shoulders), you are not going to get very far – optimal positioning allows for a good range of motion and increased performance.

Not only can poor posture impact movement and performance, but it can also be an aesthetic problem. Many individuals will have goals to improve their slouched and rounded posture in exchange for a prouder, more confident stance – humans like to be symmetrical.

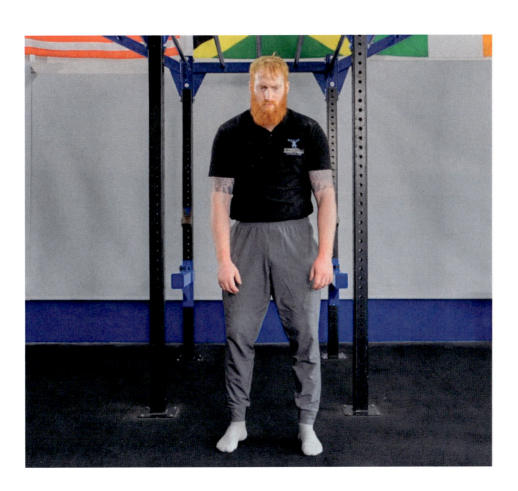

ASSESSING POSTURE

An individual's posture can be observed as soon as they walk through the door. How do they hold themselves; do they look confident or worried? Do they slouch and hold their head down?

We should also be observing both static and dynamic postures throughout a session to ensure optimal positioning. However, a static assessment of posture during a consultation or the start of a session is often used to get a good overview.

What's the first thing you are going to do when I tell you I am going to assess your posture?

Probably stand up straight and pull your head and shoulders back. Therefore, to get a more accurate reading, tell the individual to jog on the spot for a few seconds before telling them to "stop." From there, they will usually fall into their natural posture.

We can assess posture from the side and from the front and back.

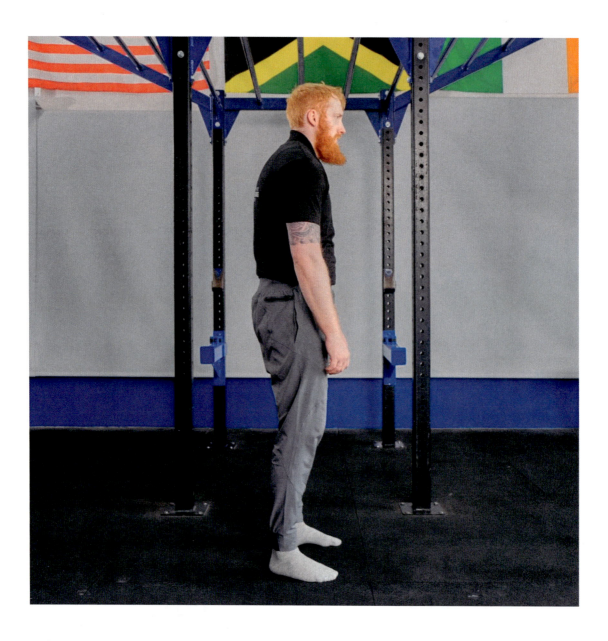

SIDE-ON VIEW

From a side-on view, we imagine a plumb line that should drop through:

- The earlobe.

- The centre of the shoulder.

- The centre of the hip.

- Slightly anterior to the midline of the knee.

- Slightly anterior to the ankle bone (malleolus).

- This allows us to clearly see if an individual has forward head posture or rounded shoulders.

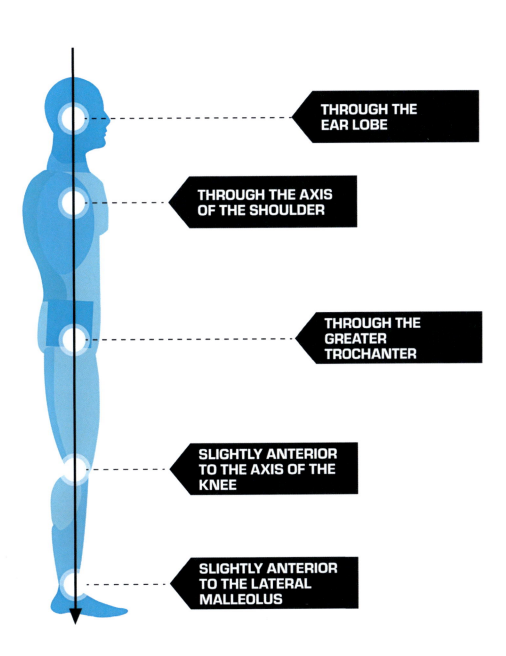

FRONT/BACK VIEW

When viewing posture from the front or back, we imagine two horizontal lines parallel to the floor:

- Between the shoulders.

- Between the hips.

This allows us to clearly see whether one shoulder or hip is higher than the other.

Although an asymmetry can be quite clear, it is not always as clear what the root cause is. The right trapezius might be considerably more developed, causing a higher shoulder, but it could also be caused by scoliosis or an imbalance at the hips.

It is essential that we have a deep understanding of how an individual muscle may impact on a structure, but also how the muscles and structures of the body work together as one big kinetic chain.

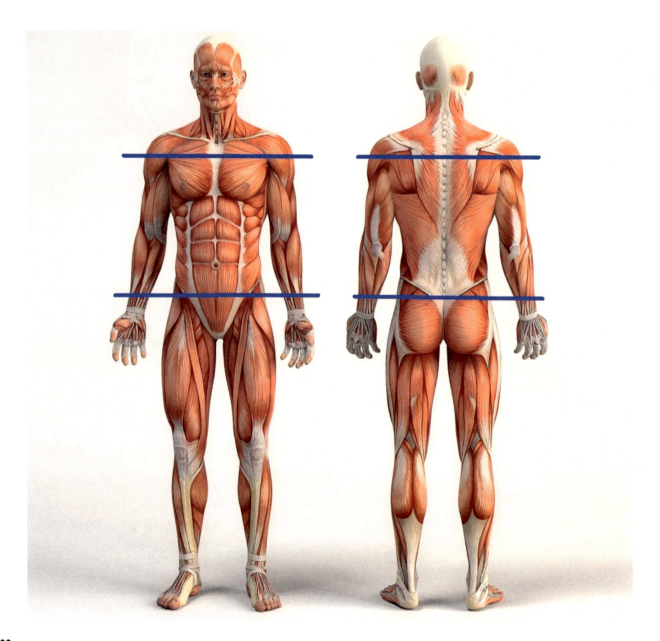

THE SPINE & PELVIS

The pelvis is made up between the sacrum and the ilium, creating the sacroiliac joints at either side of the sacrum. Therefore, pelvic positioning will impact the spine. Specifically, the lumbar spine – an anterior (forward) tilt will exaggerate the lordotic curve.

The pelvis naturally tilts forward slightly. However, there are three common ways in which the pelvis may tilt excessively:

- **Anterior Tilt:** Tilted forwards – increases lumbar lordosis (a very common sight in gyms).

- **Posterior Tilt:** Tilted backwards – causes the lumbar spine to flatten.

- **Lateral Tilt:** Tilted to one side with one ilium being higher than the other.

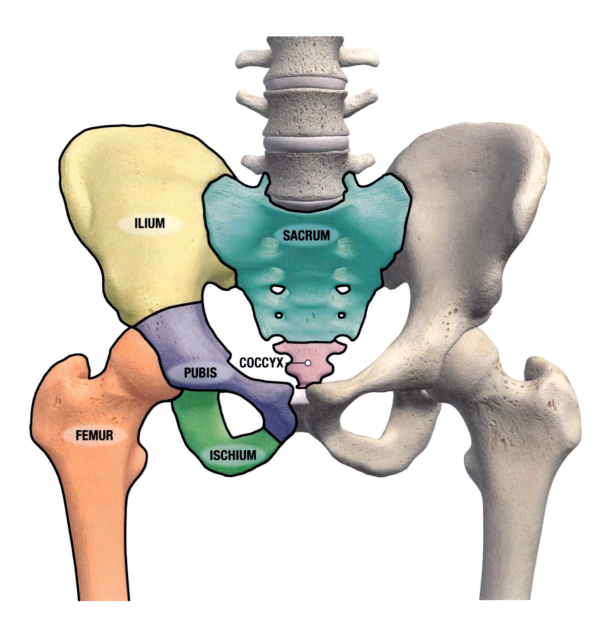

ASSESSING A LATERAL PELVIC TILT

Note: We will look at anterior and posterior pelvic tilts in the following pages when we look in more depth at standing postures.

In this section, we will look at how we assess and work to fix a lateral pelvic tilt.

The diagram below shows the Anterior Superior Iliac Spine (ASIS). These bony prominences can be used to assess pelvic positioning.

One of the easiest ways to assess pelvic positioning is to find the ASIS and hold a string or thin resistance band from one to the other. This should be done while standing barefoot in a hip-width stance in front of a mirror or the assessor. In this position, the string should be parallel to the floor. If it is not, there is a lateral pelvic tilt.

You can also place your thumbs or hands on the top of your iliac crest (edge of the ilium) to see if one is noticeably higher.

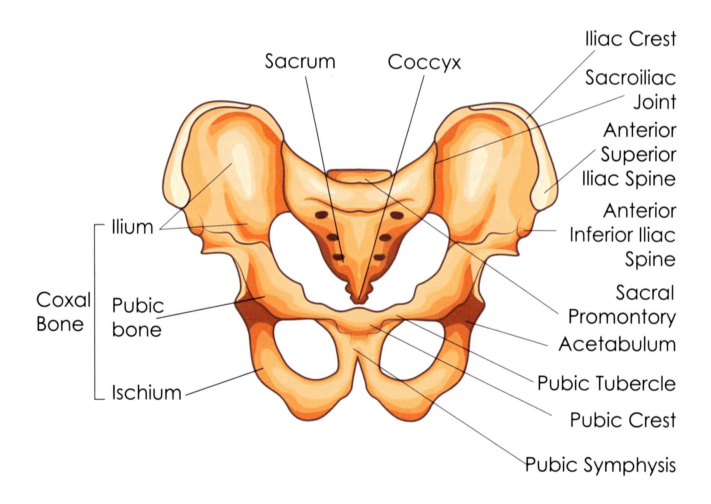

FIXING A LATERAL TILT

Lateral pelvic tilts can be caused by several things, for example:

- **Difference in Leg length:** Leg length is commonly measured by measuring the distance between the ASIS and medial malleolus (the bony prominence on the inner side of the ankle). This is done on both sides while lying flat.

- **Scoliosis:** Sideways curvature of the spine.

- **Muscle Imbalances:** This could be caused by always leaning to one side. For example, standing with most of your weight on your right leg.

The exercises in this section are not designed to fix issues caused by the top 2 bullet points. Therefore, if you think you could be experiencing problems as a result of your posture, you should see a professional who can do a full assessment. However, if we can feel clear muscle imbalances, there's lots we can do.

We refer to the high hip as a "Hip Hike" and the low hip as a "Hip Drop":

- The pelvis will show a hip hike to the side of relative weak gluteus medius, tight QL and tight adductors.

- The pelvis will show a hip drop to the side of relative tight gluteus medius, weak QL and weak adductors.

Remember, weak muscles can also become tense – every muscle wants to work (move)

We can help correct the imbalance with gluteus medius, QL and adductor strength and flexibility exercises:

- Glute release and stretch, and side-lying hip abductions.

- QL release and stretch, and hip hikes.

- Adductor release and stretch, and band adductions (opposing sides).

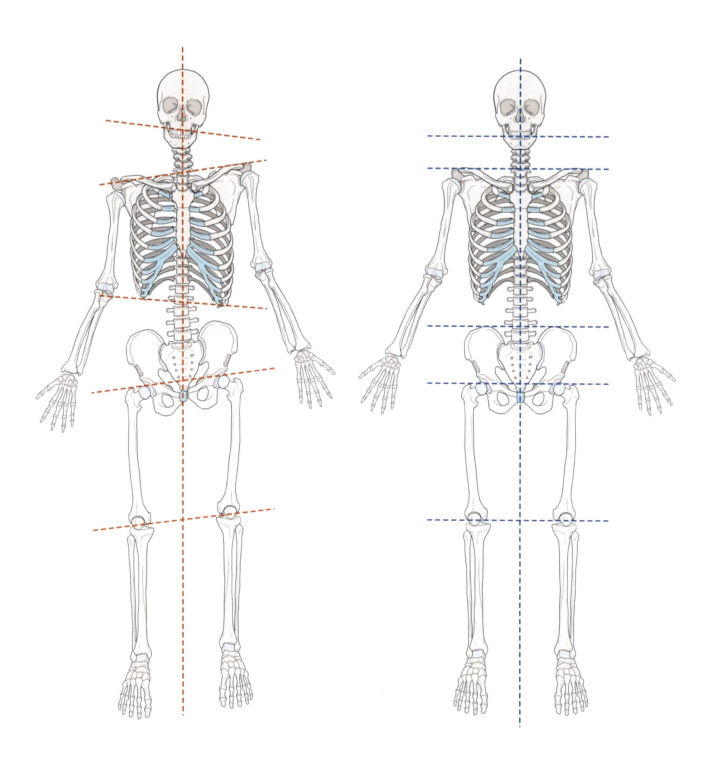

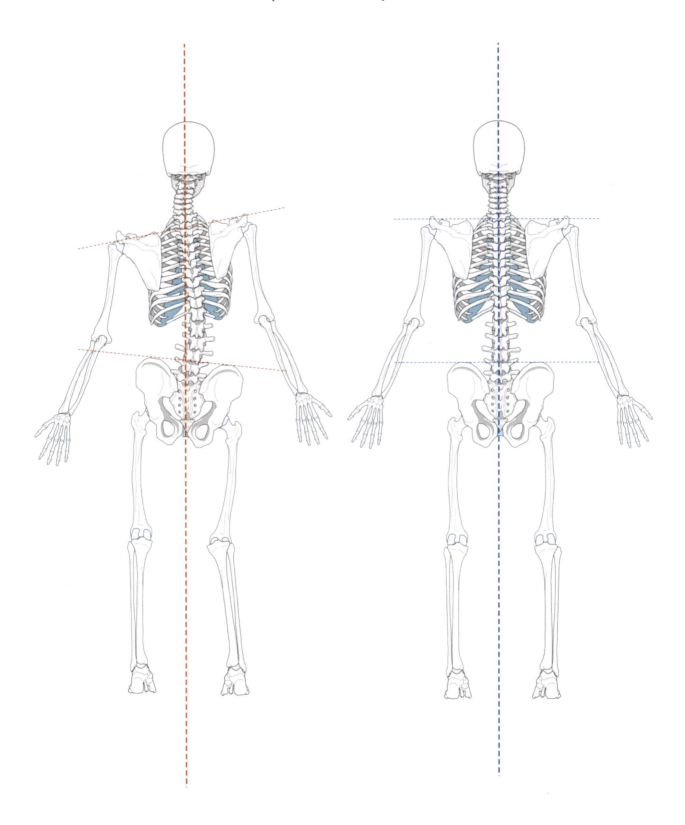

STANDING POSTURES

Standing posture types:

- Hyper-lordosis aka lordosis: Exaggerated curve of the lower (lumbar) spine and an anteriorly tilted pelvis.

- Hyper-kyphosis aka kyphosis: Exaggerated curve of the upper (thoracic) spine – kyphosis and lordosis are often present at the same time.

- Sway back: The pelvis has a posterior tilt; the hips are shifted forward, and the shoulders are shifted back. This usually results in a protracted head.

- Flat back: A flattening of the lumbar curve with a posterior pelvic tilt.

- Scoliosis: When viewed from the rear, we see an "S" or "C" shaped curve – scoliosis is more often than not a genetic trait and may require treatments such as surgery or bracing.

Rounding of the upper back and shoulders (hyper-kyphosis) and anterior pelvic tilts with exaggerated curvature of the lumbar spine (hyper-lordosis) are the most commonly seen and dealt with in a gym environment.

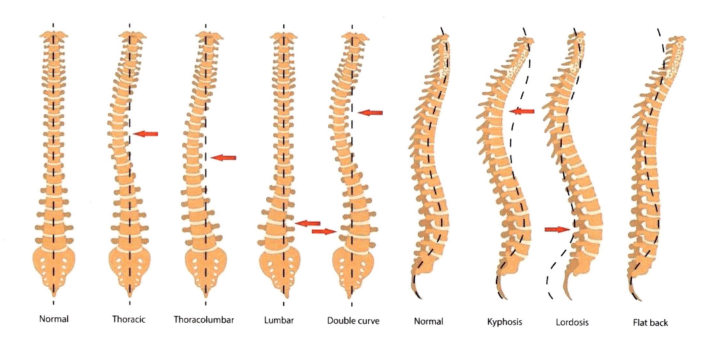

Normal   Thoracic   Thoracolumbar   Lumbar   Double curve   Normal   Kyphosis   Lordosis   Flat back

HYPER-LORDOSIS

Hyper-lordosis is usually characterized by an anteriorly tilted pelvis and an exaggerated curve of the lower spine

The relationship between the muscles that surround these areas is often referred to as lower crossed syndrome:

- Tight / Shortened erector spinae and quadratus lumborum (QL's)
- Tight / shortened iliopsoas (psoas major and iliacus).
- Weak / lengthened abdominals.
- Weak / lengthened gluteals and hamstrings.

We can help correct these issues with:

- QL release and stretches.
- The couch stretch (hip flexors and quadriceps).
- Glute Bridges and Hamstring Curls.
- Abdominal Crunches.

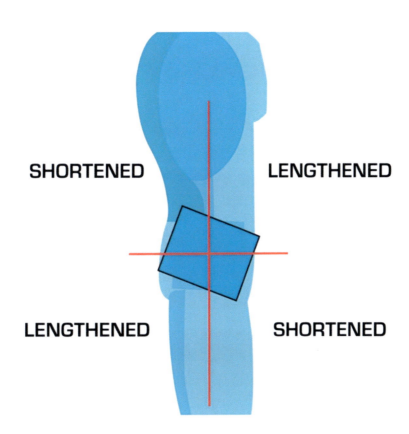

HYPER-KYPHOSIS

Hyper-kyphosis is usually characterized by a rounded upper back, rounded shoulders, and forward head posture.

The relationship between the muscles that surround these areas is often referred to as upper crossed syndrome:

- Tight / shortened pectorals.

- Tight / shortened upper trapezius and levator scapula.

- Weak / lengthened deep neck flexors.

- Weak / lengthened lower trapezius, rhomboids and serratus anterior.

We can help correct these issues with:

- Pec release and stretch.

- Trap and levator scapula release and stretch.

- Neck flexor strength exercise.

- Band horizontal Pulls.

- Palms forward, bent over lateral raises.

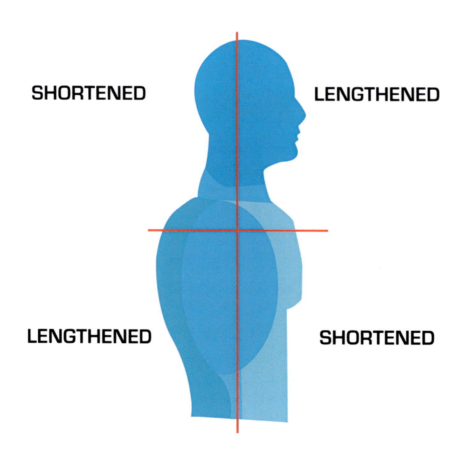

THE FEET

When it comes to corrective exercise, we have what is often referred to as the domino effect. For example, an over pronated foot on one side can cause the knee on that side to fall inwards (knee valgus). This may lead to an imbalanced squat where the weight is shifted to one side, putting excess stress on the joints and leading to strength imbalances.

Due to the fact our feet are the first point of contact with the ground. It is clear to see why it is essential to have strong and stable feet and ankles.

An individual's foot may:

Pronate: This means the ankle is everting slightly. During overpronation, much of the weight is transferred to the inner side of the ball of the foot due to a lack of arch.

Supinate: This means the ankle is inverting slightly with more weight on the outer side of the foot – inversion sprains are the most common form of ankle sprain.

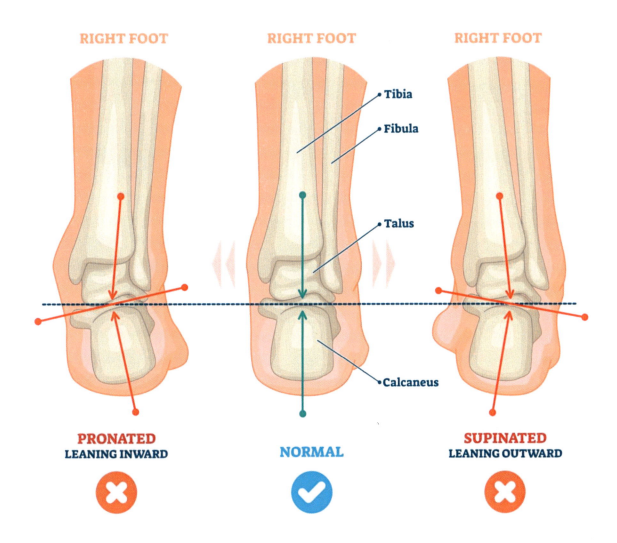

TRAINING BRACE: CORE DEVELOPMENT

Brace is the ability to isometrically contact muscles (no change in muscle length) and create tension. This helps us to stabilize positioning, movement and resist external forces. When this is performed throughout the entire body, we refer to it as total body tension – we use total body tension when we lift weights.

When we resistance train, especially with free weights and compound movements that involve multiple joints and muscle groups, we are under tension (time under tension refers to how long you are under load). Therefore, muscles are bracing and working isometrically to support the action. During a heavy squat or deadlift, the trunk muscles have to work exceptionally hard to maintain the optimal positioning and support the lower back.

Some coaches and athletes will argue that large compound movements such as the squat or deadlift are more than enough development for the trunk muscles and that specific isometric holds like a plank are a waste of time. However, it fundamentally comes down to what level the individual is at, what they need, and what their preferences are.

We should always prioritize compound movements that elicit the greatest response. However, if there is time to add in isolation work or specific trunk strengthening or stability exercises, it has its benefits – the argument that you could just do more squats is redundant as there is an optimal amount of volume for any movement.

Before we look at how we can specifically train brace, we will look at how we use breathing techniques correctly - applying the right breathing techniques will reduce your risk of injury and improve performance.

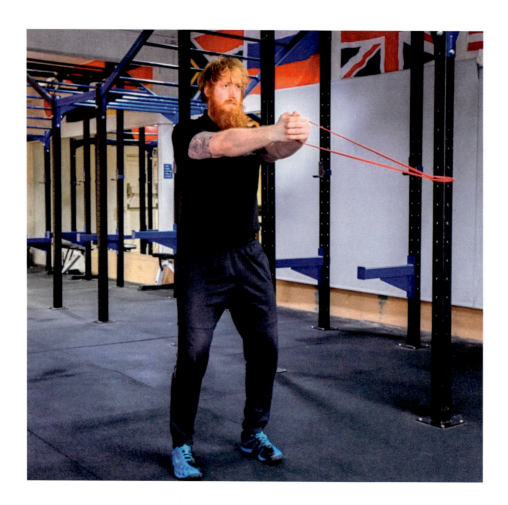

BREATHING

It is important to breathe deeply "through your belly" using your diaphragm. This pulls your diaphragm down, expands your lungs, and allows you to take in more oxygen.

To practice diaphragmatic breathing, place one hand on your chest and one on your belly. Imagine a balloon in your stomach. As you inhale through your nose or mouth, the balloon expands, and as you exhale through your mouth, it deflates. If your chest raises instead of your belly, your breathing is too shallow.

Many people breathe through the top of their chest, especially when mouth-breathing. This causes muscles that are not designed for respiration to overwork and create excess tension in the neck muscles. Breathing at the top of the chest can also weaken the diaphragm through underuse and result in fatigue during exercise and a performance reduction.

Nasal breathing increases rib cage and diaphragm engagement during inhalation. This is beneficial because it drives more oxygen into your lungs' lower lobes compared to mouth breathing. However, nasal breathing may not allow you to draw in enough oxygen when working at a high intensity. Whether you use nasal or mouth breathing, the important thing is to maintain a constant rhythm, rather than randomly mixing the two.

During resistance training, we use a biomechanical breathing style that maximizes performance and minimizes injury risk.

When using biomechanical breathing, you match your inhalation with the exercise's eccentric (downward) phase and your exhalation with the concentric (upward) phase. Most lifters inhale during the start of the eccentric phase and exhale during the latter stage of the concentric phase (concentric exhalation).

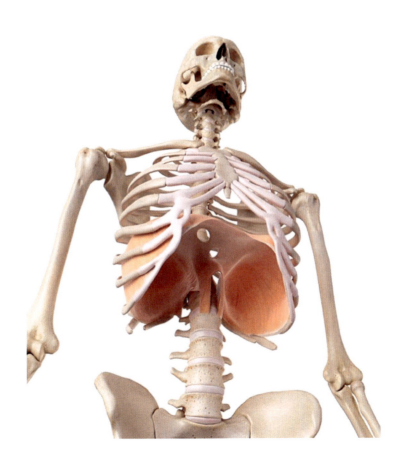

THE VALSALVA MANOEUVRE

Biomechanical breathing is often coupled with the use of the Valsalva manoeuvre, which is "a moderately forceful attempted exhalation against a closed airway" (like equalizing your ears on an airplane by blowing against a pinched nose).

This manoeuvre, combined with braced trunk muscles, creates intra-abdominal pressure (IAP) and stabilizes the spine. To visualize this, imagine the rigidity of a sealed plastic bottle full of air compared to an open bottle.

Using the Valsalva manoeuvre can cause a rise in blood pressure and dizziness. However, the performance benefits and reduced risk of injury generally outweigh the risks, barring other health considerations.

Bracing and creating tension is a good thing when lifting heavy, and the benefits are emphasized with a weightlifting belt – a weightlifting belt gives the lifter something to push their belly against, creating even more tension and maximizing intra-abdominal pressure.

However, during other forms of movement and physical training, excessive tension will cause fatigue and reduced speed and mobility.

The force-velocity paradox: Ultimately, we need to produce force to create movement and speed. However, the corresponding tension that is created restricts speed. Therefore, there needs to be a balance between contraction and relaxation phases. Athletic performance is not just about the ability to produce force quickly (rate of force development). It's also about how fast a muscle can contract, relax (to maximize joint velocity), and re-contract – we often call this a double pulse.

When there is no need to create maximal total body tension, we instead aim to regulate our breathing in an optimal way for the activity we are doing – anatomical breathing.

For example, while running, an individual may inhale for three strides and exhale for three strides.

We can also consider the position of the body. For example, during a kettlebell swing, we could exhale at the bottom of the movement while the body is bent over and inhale at the top of the movement while the torso is upright.

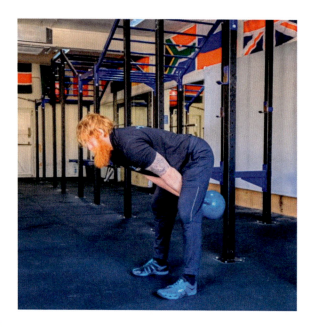 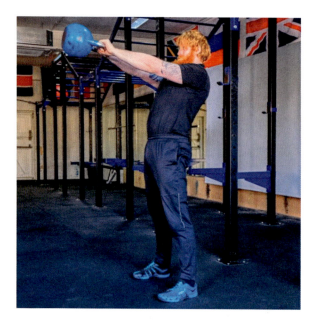

ANTI-MOVEMENTS

Anti-movements are the best way to classify brace training. We put trunk bracing into four categories:

- **Anti-Extension:** Resisting the spine extending (primarily engaging the rectus abdominis), i.e., A front plank.

- **Anti-Flexion:** Resisting the spine flexing (primarily engaging the erector spinae), i.e., A dorsal raise hold.

- **Anti-Lateral Flexion:** Resisting the spine flexing to the side (primarily engaging the obliques and QL's unilaterally), i.e., A unilateral loaded carry (walking with a dumbbell or kettlebell in one hand).

- **Anti-Rotation:** Resisting the spine rotating (primarily engaging the obliques and QL's), i.e., A Pallof press.

Note: Some exercises will target multiple categories. For example, anti-rotation and anti-lateral flexion are usually worked concurrently.

Anti-Extension	Anti-Flexion	Anti-Lateral Flexion	Anti-Rotation
Front Plank	Dorsal Raise Holds	Side Plank	Paloff Variations
Ab Roll Out	Hinge Holds	Suitcase Carry	Birddog
Dead Bug	Ball Slams		

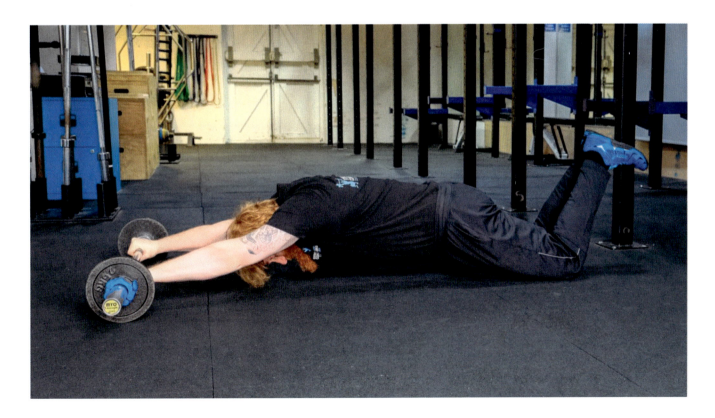

ROTATION

Rotation is primarily facilitated through the hip and shoulder joints (ball and sockets) and the spine via a series of facet joints.

Most of the exercises we perform in the gym involve flexing and extending the joints, forwards and backwards (up and down) and in some occasions side to side (sagittal and frontal planes). However, the one plane of movement that often gets left out is the transverse plane, or rotational movements.

Our training should prioritise movements that take us forward and back, up and down. However, in many daily activities and sporting movements we perform rotation or couple it with other movements.

Torque is a rotational force that can be quite stressful and therefore, not only is it essential that we add in rotational movements to help develop rotational strength and build performance, but also so we can accommodate the huge stress that rotation can put on the body.

Not only is it essential that we build rotational strength, we need to ensure we have the mobility to rotate fully without having to compensate.

One of the most common movement limitations we see is a lack of thoracic rotation, and just like with thoracic extension, if there is an inability to perform the action, other areas might compensate, for example the lower spine.

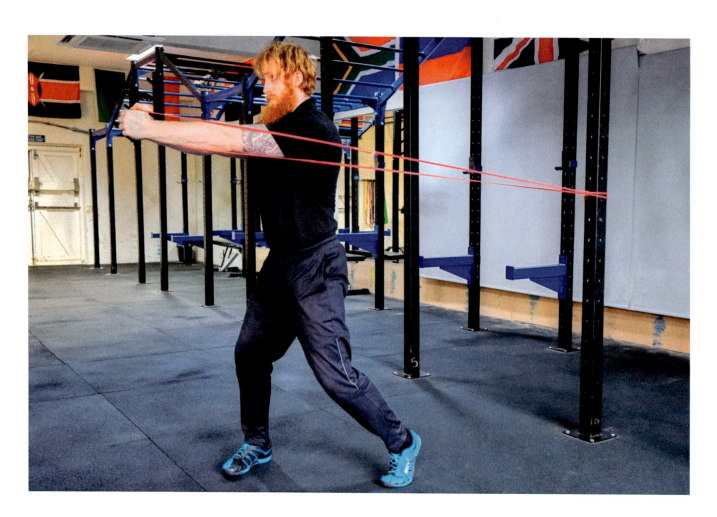

MOBILITY AND FLEXIBILITY

Now we have covered the fundamentals of posture and movement. We will look at how we develop mobility and flexibility before delving into each joint action. We will work these muscles and movement in isolation with strength and mobility exercises before progressing onto the best compound exercises for the lower and upper body. We will also look at more of the common issues listed in the corrective exercise section throughout all of this.

It's vital to understand the difference between flexibility and mobility. Flexibility is the muscle's ability to lengthen, so a test for this would be lying flat on your back while a partner lifts your leg to test hamstring flexibility (passive stretch).

On the other hand, mobility refers to a joint's ability to move through its full range of motion (ROM). Therefore, not only does it involve muscle flexibility but also joint structure, motor control, and stability.

There are many misconceptions about both flexibility and mobility and the techniques used to progress them. People often perceive flexibility to be the fundamental factor when it comes to injury prevention. Yes, having good flexibility is key and can prevent muscle strains. However, we must find the optimal balance between joint mobility and stability. We want our muscles to lengthen, but we also want a certain amount of muscle tension (tone) and the ability to contact our muscles forcefully.

The key to injury prevention is better described as "having strength through a full ROM." And, of course, load management (good programming).

An example of how excessive ROM can be detrimental is hypermobility, which is often misnomered as being "double-jointed," suggesting there is more than one joint. In actuality, it means the ligaments that attach bone to bone and support the joint are laxer, allowing for a greater ROM. Now, this can make for a great party trick. However, it can also make the joint more prone to subluxation (partial dislocation) and dislocation (the shoulder joint, for example).

This being said, having limited ROM can drastically reduce performance, and this is all too apparent when you watch someone try to perform an overhead squat without sufficient mobility – I have personally seen lifters who can strictly press over 100kg, tremble under a 20kg overhead squat.

We can take a holistic approach to mobility and work the entire body. However, the training principal individuality is always present. Person 'A' may find their hip flexors and quadriceps feel tight or tense, whereas person 'B' finds their calves and hamstrings are tight or tense. Therefore, it makes sense for people to take an individualized approach. However, is stretching always the answer?

We hear terms like shortened, lengthened, tight, tense, lax, inactive, hypotonic (abnormally low muscle tone), overactive, and hypertonic (abnormally high muscle tone), and these terms are often thrown around haphazardly. But what does it actually mean when a muscle is tight or tense? Does it mean that the muscle's resting length is shorter than it should be or that the muscle is permanently contracted?

In actuality, for the most part, when your muscle feels tight or tense, there is no measurable, mechanical explanation for that feeling. The muscle has the same resting length as it did before you felt the excess tension. However, this does not mean the sensation isn't there, it is just far more complex than what is perceived, and it can be helped with the right techniques.

There are various theories as to why stretching increases flexibility such as viscoelastic deformation, plastic deformation, increased sarcomeres in series, and neuromuscular relaxation. However, Stretching does not primarily develop flexibility by changing the muscle's mechanical properties and making it longer on a structural level. Instead, we increase our stretch tolerance, which is sensory (neuromuscular).

This can be illustrated when holding a stretch for a moderate amount of time. Initially, when you apply the stretch, you feel tension within the muscle. However, as the stretch is held, this tension reduces, and you can gradually increase the ROM.

We can also illustrate the nervous system's incredible nature by using muscle energy techniques, which capitalize on mechanisms such as post-isometric relaxation or reciprocal inhibition to produce a much greater ROM in a short space of time – these will be covered in far more detail.

On top of this, we don't even have to target the muscle directly to increase its flexibility. Simply rolling the soles of your feet or massaging your sub-occipitals (muscles on the back of your head) can release your hamstrings – note, these are all short-term neurological adaptations.

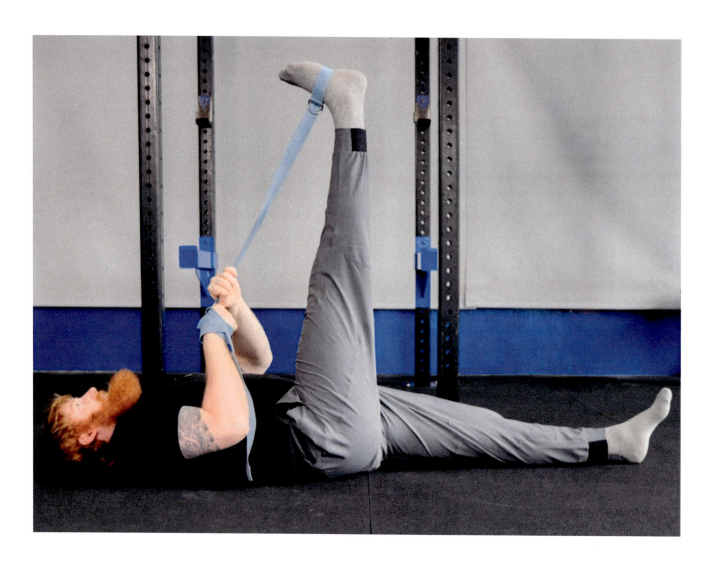

RELEASE TECHNIQUES

Release techniques are a method of hands-on therapy that you can perform yourself, usually with a foam roller or massage ball. These techniques use pressure to result in a short-term release of muscle tension, which in turn can allow you to achieve a more effective stretch or a full ROM squat, which of course, can then result in long-term adaptations over consistent training.

Since this is a neuromuscular response, the mechanisms by which rolling or kneading a muscle with a roller or ball can be quite complicated and debated by leading scientists.

A common explanation is that applying pressure to a muscle stimulates a proprioceptor known as the Golgi tendon organ, which responds to changes in muscle tension and inhibits the muscle to ensure damage is not caused.

Note: Muscle spindles are a proprioceptor that responds to changes in muscle length. When a muscle lengthens, they send a signal to the spinal cord that then innovates an involuntary contraction in the muscle.

For example, suppose you roll onto the outer side of your ankle (an action that can cause an inversion sprain). In that case, the peroneal muscles will lengthen, the muscle spindles will detect this and cause them to contract, pulling the ankle back and hopefully preventing an inversion sprain (the most common type of ankle sprain).

Another reasoning as to why release techniques can be so effective is Diffuse Noxious Inhibitory Control (DNIC), which is one of several varieties of "descending modulation," where the brain adjusts the amount of nociception (the perception or sensation of pain) – the brain inhibits nociceptive signals from traveling up the spinal cord to the brain.

DNIC is triggered by a sustained nociceptive input, for example, applying pressure to the muscle. This can actually suppress nociception not just from the local area but also from distant regions. Therefore, if your right hip is sore and you roll the quadriceps on your left leg, the DNIC will reduce the discomfort in both the quadriceps and the hip – this makes a lot of sense why rolling a muscle can feel so good.

On top of all of this, rolling a muscle will encourage blood flow and increase deep muscle temperature, and a warm muscle is a more pliable muscle.

Release techniques are going to feel a little uncomfortable, and some areas are inherently more tender than others. However, there is a clear line between "a good hurt" and outright pain that can cause trauma.

When it comes to release techniques, the key is to stimulate, not annihilate. Yes, you want to knead the muscle, but you don't want to cause unnecessary trauma, i.e., bruising.

You can roll a muscle for 20-30 seconds or even 2-3 minutes. However, for most large muscle masses (the quadriceps, for example), I tend to recommend 30-60 seconds of faster-paced rolling for warm-ups and 1-2 minutes of slower-paced rolling during cooldowns or recovery sessions.

Yes, you can roll muscles before a workout to increase circulation and muscle pliability. However, you don't want to relax the muscles too much before a session. You want some tension in the muscles.

STRETCHING

When we think of stretching, we tend to think of someone statically holding a position for a short period to apply a stretch to a specific muscle. However, there are many forms of stretching.

This e-book will concentrate on static stretches as a whole. However, we will also introduce more advanced forms of stretching that are listed in the table in the next slide – I will introduce some of my favourite PNF drills.

Static	Dynamic	Proprioceptive Neuromuscular Facilitation (PNF)
Active: The body part is moved into position and is actively held in the static position using the surrounding musculature.	Controlled Dynamic: Actively moving through a joint's full range of motion in a controlled, fluid manner.	Contract-Relax: This is also known as post-isometric relaxation (PIR) and capitalizes on muscle inhibition.
Passive: The body part is moved into position and held there using a supporting structure such as a wall or a partner.	Ballistic: Using momentum and often a jerking action to increase the range of a dynamic stretch.	Contract-Relax Agonist Contraction: Actively engaging the antagonist (opposing muscle) during the stretch to capitalize on reciprocal inhibition.
Maintenance: Short stretches held for 10-30 seconds.		
Developmental: Longer stretches held for 1-2 minutes (usually for multiple sets).		

Stretching can feel uncomfortable, but just as with the release techniques, it should only be a reasonable level of discomfort, not a painful experience. If the muscle starts to tremble, your breathing starts to speed up, or you feel forced to hold your breath, ease off a little.

The "barrier" position is a term used to describe the point at which the muscle first experiences the sensation of tightness during a stretch. This point is important as we use it during PNF stretches. It also a great illustration of how a prolonged stretch teaches the muscle to tolerate greater extension (not make the muscle fibres longer) – numerous barrier positions may be experienced.

For the most part, when people hold stretches for short periods on an irregular basis, the adaptations made are short-term, acting like a "muscle release." However, with regular developmental stretches, long-term adaptations will be made.

OSCILLATORY AND BALLISTIC STRETCHES

Oscillatory stretching is a great way to turn many of the static stretches within this book into dynamic stretches. Therefore, it acts as a great way to warm the muscles and build stretch tolerance before training.

To perform an oscillatory stretch, you move through the full or a partial range of the stretch in a smooth and fluid motion (oscillations). For example, during the frog stretch, you can move your hips forward and back.

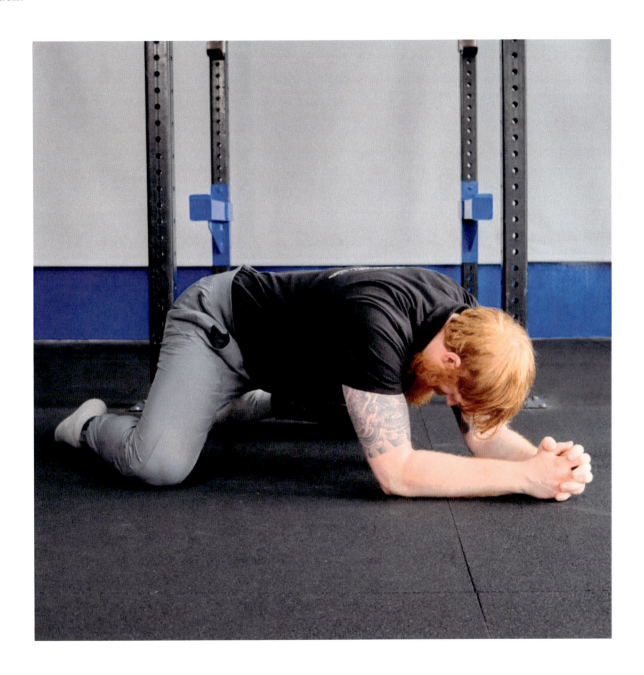

Ballistic stretches are similar to oscillatory stretches in the sense that you repeatedly move in and out of the end range position. However, as the name suggests, during ballistic stretches, this is done with much more momentum.

There are three phases to a ballistic stretch:

- Initial Phase: The antagonist muscle performs concentric action to initiate the action.

- Coasting Phase: The momentum gained from the initial phase allows the stretch to be taken beyond the normal range.

- Deceleration Phase: This is initiated by eccentric actions of the agonist (stretched muscle) as the muscle passes its normal ROM.

Ballistic stretches are sometimes used by athletes. For example, it isn't uncommon to see a gymnast bend forward to stretch their hamstrings and back and use a bouncing/jerky action to increase the range of motion. There is no doubt that using bounces at the end range can help to increase the stretch tolerance of a muscle. However, it is clear to see how ballistic stretching is often seen as dangerous.

Ballistic stretches do have a higher risk of muscle and tendon strains and even ligament sprains. Therefore, they should only be used by well-trained individuals that know what they are doing.

On top of this, the explosive eccentric stretch is likely to invoke the stretch reflex (involuntary contraction of the muscle), which in essence is exciting the muscle rather than relaxing it. This is arguably good during a warm-up, specifically the potentiation phase, where we aim to prime the muscles for maximal intensity. However, if the aim to relax the muscle and ease tension, then ballistic stretching is not the way to go.

An example of where ballistic stretching is used to great effect in strength training is using pulses during a squat. During a pulse, the lifter reaches the bottom of the squat and proceeds to perform a secondary bounce (pulse) of 3-6 inches. When working with weight, a lifter may perform 1-3 pulses per rep. However, prior to a squat session, a lifter may perform 5-10 pulses in a deep bodyweight squat to help prepare for the session.

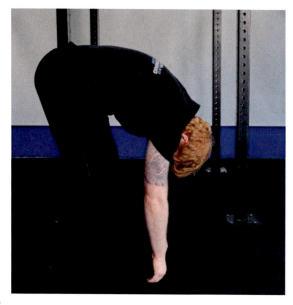 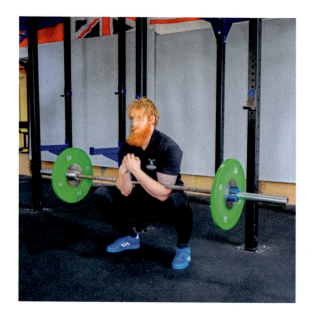

LOADED STRETCHES

Loaded stretches are by far the most unheard-of and underrated way of developing flexibility and are especially good pre training session. However, in my experience, they are the most effective for many muscle groups.

Loaded stretches involve holding a weight at a muscle's end range of motion. Essentially this is just a pause or isometric hold at the bottom of a movement. However, the emphasis is on the stretch in the muscle. Therefore, the appropriate loads (low-moderate) should be used when pushing the end range.

Some of my favourite loaded stretches include:

- The Overhead Squat – absolute favourite!
- Lying Lat Stretch.
- Dumbbell Fly Stretch.

One of the best examples of loaded stretching is the overhead squat with a barbell. I have worked with literally dozens of clients with terrible mobility that had spent months doing the same stretching regimes to no prevail. After a couple of weeks of overhead squat work (starting with regressions), their mobility in their lower body, shoulders, and thoracic spine improved dramatically.

To regress the overhead squat, I have the lifter stand with their heels on plates. From there, they use a technique barbell (5-10kg) and overhead squat as deep as possible. This is pushed until they achieve a decent ROM. From there, we progressively load the weight, and within a few sessions, most people are achieving a decent overhead squat.

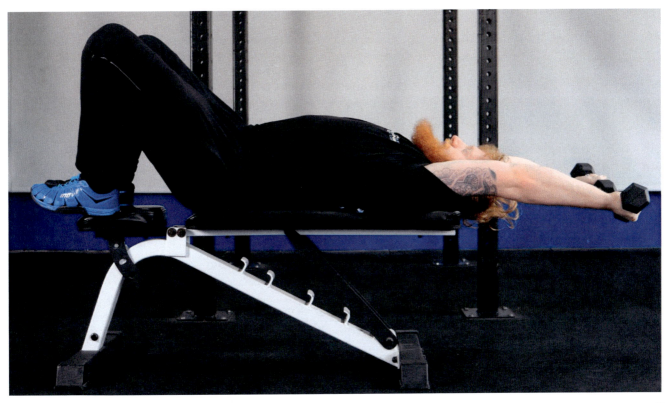

PROPRIOCEPTIVE NEUROMUSCULAR FACILITATION (PNF)

This section will look at PNF (proprioceptive neuromuscular facilitation) stretches in a little more detail.

PNF stretches essentially capitalize on neuromuscular mechanisms that elicit relaxation (inhibition) in the muscle and allow us to achieve a greater stretch.

Note: PNF techniques commonly come under the category of Muscle Energy Techniques (MET), a term used to describe a range of physical therapy techniques.

Two fundamental principles of PNF:

Post-Isometric Relaxation (PIR): Following a contraction (6-8 seconds – 50-60% of maximal contraction), a muscle enters a deeper state of relaxation (for around 5 seconds). These contractions are usually isometric (no change in muscle length – pushing against a partner or an object) but can also be performed with a concentric contraction (muscle shortening).

Reciprocal Inhibition (RI): When a muscle contracts, the opposing muscle must relax to allow for efficient movement. Therefore, when contracting an opposing muscle or directly after, you are able to achieve a greater stretch. The nature of this technique allows you to engage the opposing muscles to "actively" reach the barrier position of the targeted muscle.

Note: A contraction of just 20-30% is usually sufficient to invoke the desired response. However, clients will often try to push maximally – the most intuitive cue is to instruct them to contact at 50-60%.

Both methods can be performed with or without a partner, and ultimately, it comes down to being quite creative in how you apply a contraction of the agonist or antagonist – in this book, I will introduce some of my favourite.

One of the most common PNF stretches is the lying hamstrings variation with a partner.

During this stretch, the client lies down, and the coach kneels in a position where they can take one of the client's legs and raise it into a hamstring stretch.

During a PIR stretch, once the barrier position is met, the client can push against the coach's hand or shoulder with their leg to contract their hamstring isometrically (could also be done concentrically if the coach allows the leg to be pushed towards the floor).

This contraction is held for 6-8 seconds and following a 1-2 second period to allow the muscle to relax fully, the coach instructs the client to exhale (after a big deep breath during the 1-2 second period) and increases the stretch to reach the next barrier position – this process is usually performed 3 times.

Note: Prior to contracting the muscle, the coach can ease off from the barrier position slightly to ensure that it is not too uncomfortable, and the muscle doesn't start to tremble.

Each barrier position is commonly held for 5-10 seconds, but 15-20 seconds will better allow for the neuromuscular system to adapt to the new length.

The final barrier position should be held for at least 20-30 seconds and can be held for 1-minute if the muscle is particularly tense – note, the entire drill may take 2-3 minutes. Therefore, some positions may become uncomfortable.

To perform the same hamstring stretch from a lying position using the RI method, rather than pushing the leg down toward the floor to engage the hamstrings, the client would pull their leg up towards themselves and push their knee into extension (the coach can hold the client's shin back) to engage the hip flexors and quadriceps.

Another RI hamstring stretch variation involves the client raising a straight leg by contracting their hip flexors and quadriceps. From there, once the barrier position is met, the coach can hold the leg to allow for a relaxed stretch before the client engages their hip flexors and quads again to reach the next barrier position.

To perform either stretch technique without a partner, the client could use a strap while lying or stand and place one heel onto a box (20 inches). On the box, they can push their heel into the box to create a hamstring contraction (PIR) or pick their leg up and contact their quadriceps (RI).

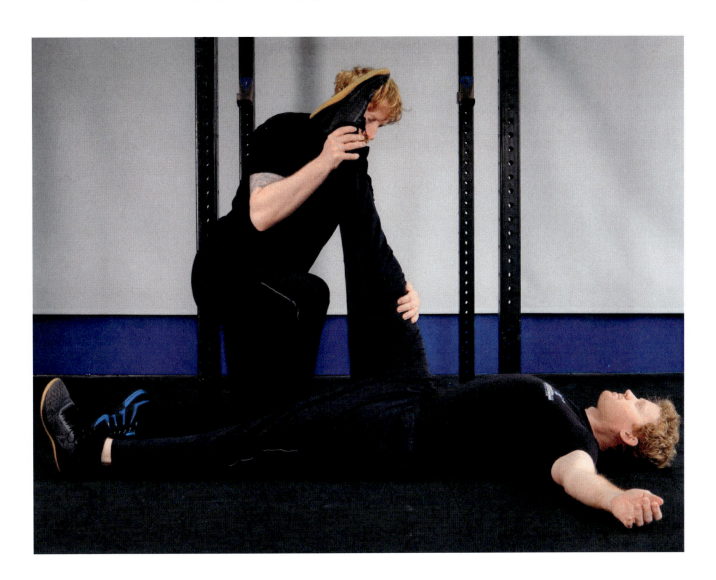

BAND DISTRACTIONS

Using resistance bands can be a highly effective way to increase the intensity of a stretch or assist a stretch by distracting a joint to allow for a greater range of motion.

The elastic nature of resistance bands means they can be used to pull you into a greater stretch passively, or you can pull/push against them to create a PNF stretch. However, caution should be practiced to ensure the band is not able to cause injury.

When you attach a resistance band to a sturdy structure, such as a post, there is essentially an endless list of ways in which you can attach the band to yourself to have it pull you into a stretch. For example, many of the conventional static stretches within this book can be performed with an anterior or posterior pull from the band (you can play with different setups and see what creates the best stretch).

Joint distraction refers to when the joint (two bones meeting to form a joint) are pulled apart slightly to create more freedom of movement.

For example, if you grab your left hand (close to the wrist) and pull it away from your forearm, this will distract the joint and allow you to achieve a greater stretch on the surrounding tissues.

One of the best examples of where bands might be used is during an ankle dorsiflexion drill. During this drill, a high-tension band is placed around the top of your foot, right in the crease of the ankle joint, to pull the talus back. From there, you stride forward onto a low box so that the band is pulling your talus back to reduce the risk of impingement and increase ankle dorsiflexion.

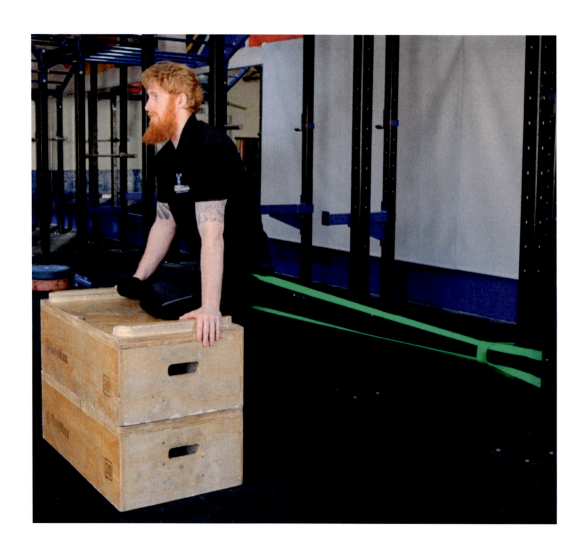

FLEXIBILITY TESTS

In this section, we will look at four popular flexibility tests:

- **Sit and Reach Test:** Hamstrings and Back.

- **Knee to Wall Test:** Calves (dorsiflexion).

- **Back Scratch Test:** Shoulders (internal and external rotators).

- **Lying Lat & Triceps Test:** Latissimus dorsi and the long head of the triceps.

Remember, it is not a case of the more flexible, the better. We are looking for the ability to work through a healthy range of motion. Restrictions in any of these areas will be very evident due to poor scores and an intense feeling of tension.

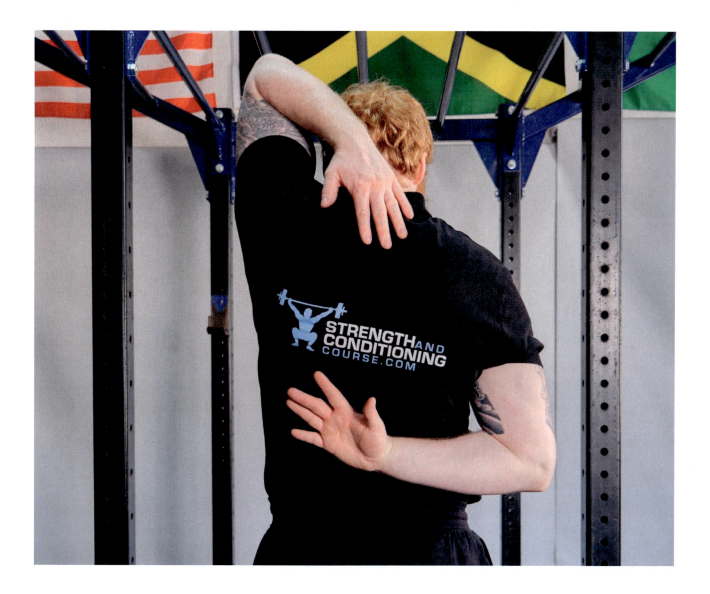

SIT AND REACH TEST

Equipment: A sit and reach box / a ruler on a step or low box.

Procedure: The athlete removes their footwear and sits on the floor with their legs stretched out to their front (legs together). The soles of the athlete's feet are placed flat against the box. Both knees should be locked and pressed flat to the floor (the assessor may assist by holding them down).

With their palms facing downwards, and their hands on top of each other or side by side, the athlete reaches forward along the measuring line as far as possible.

Ensure that the hands remain at the same level, not one reaching further forward than the other. After some practice reaches, the athlete reaches out and holds that position for 1-2 seconds (no jerking movements) while the distance is recorded.

Scoring: The score is recorded to the nearest centimeter or half inch. Some test versions use the level of the feet as the zero mark, while others have the zero mark 9 inches (23cm) before the feet. There is also a modified sit and reach test which adjusts the zero-mark depending on the arm and leg length of the subject.

MODIFIED SIT AND REACH TEST

To perform a modified sit and reach test, the athlete sits with their back and head against a wall.

A sit and reach box with an adjustable measure is used or a ruler on a box. While keeping their back and head against the wall, the athlete reaches forward to adjust the measure so that the zero mark is at their fingertips. From there, the athlete relaxes before performing the sit and reach test as per the protocol above.

Note: Some test protocols require the athlete to keep their shoulder blades retracted.

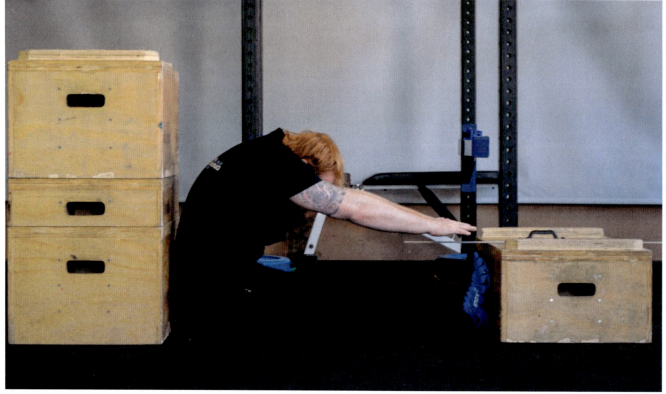

KNEE TO WALL TEST

Equipment: Wall, ruler, or tape measure.

Procedure: The athlete stands a short distance away from a wall, with one leg in front of the other. Keeping their heel of the front foot on the ground, they then try and bend at the knee and touch the knee to the wall.

If done successfully, the athlete moves further away from the wall and tries again. The athlete keeps repeating this action until they are unable to touch the wall. Measure the distance from the front of the foot to the wall at the maximum distance the knee can touch the wall. Repeat the same procedure for each leg.

Scoring: Measure the maximum distance from the toe to the wall. There are norms available for this test. However, this test is often used to compare the difference between an injured and uninjured side.

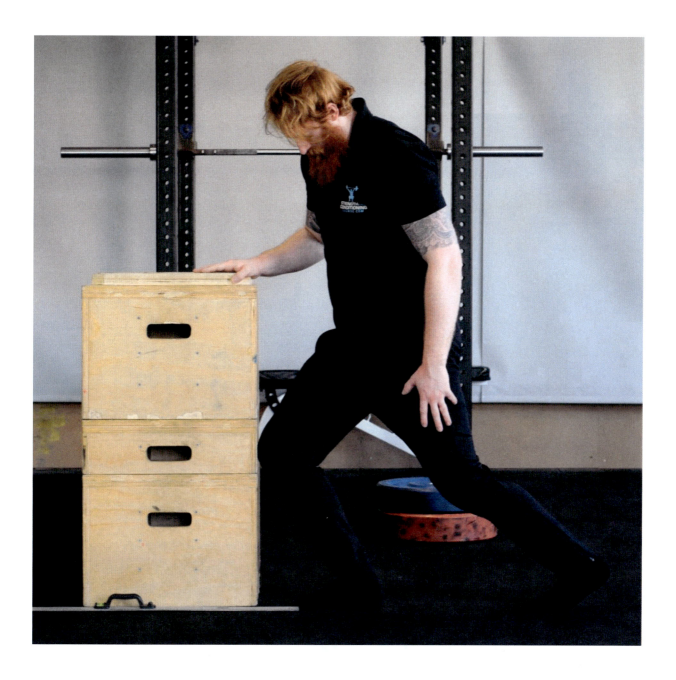

BACK SCRATCH TEST

Equipment: Ruler or tape measure.

Procedure: This test is done in a standing position. The athlete places one hand over their shoulder and behind their head and reaches as far as possible down the middle of their back (with their palm touching their body and their fingers directed downwards).

The athlete places their other arm behind their lower back (palm facing outward and fingers upward) and reaches up as far as possible, attempting to touch or overlap the middle fingers of both hands. The assessor can ensure the fingers are aligned and measure the distance between the tips of the middle fingers.

Scoring: If the fingertips touch, then the score is zero. If they do not touch, measure the distance between the fingertips (a negative score), if they overlap, measure by how much (a positive score). Practice two times, and then test two times. Stop the test if the subject experiences pain.

Record the best score to the nearest centimeter or 1/2 inch. The higher the score the better the result.

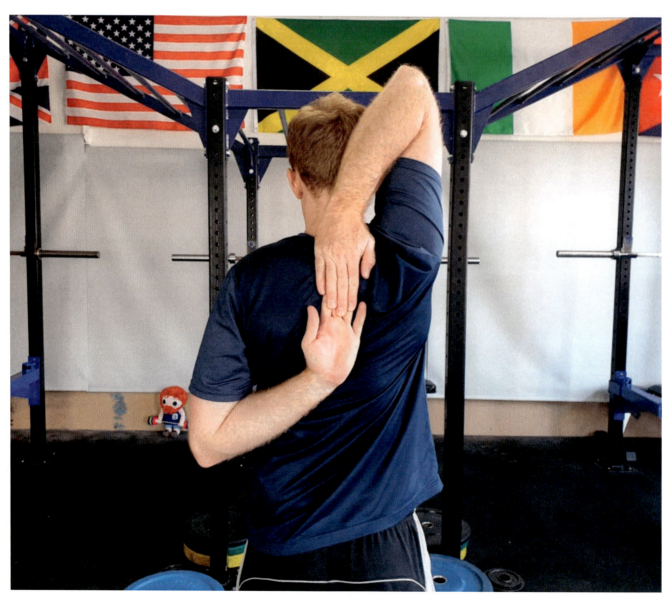

LYING LAT AND TRICEPS STRETCH

Equipment: A ruler or tape measure

Procedure: The athlete lies flat on their back with their knees bent (ensure the lower back is flat to the floor). The athlete then brings their hands to their front with their palms together. The athlete then slowly takes their arms overhead while keeping their elbows straight.

Scoring: Measure the distance between the hands and the floor. If the athlete is able to bring their hands to the floor with straight arms and without compensating by over-arching their lower spine, then they are considered to have good lat and triceps flexibility.

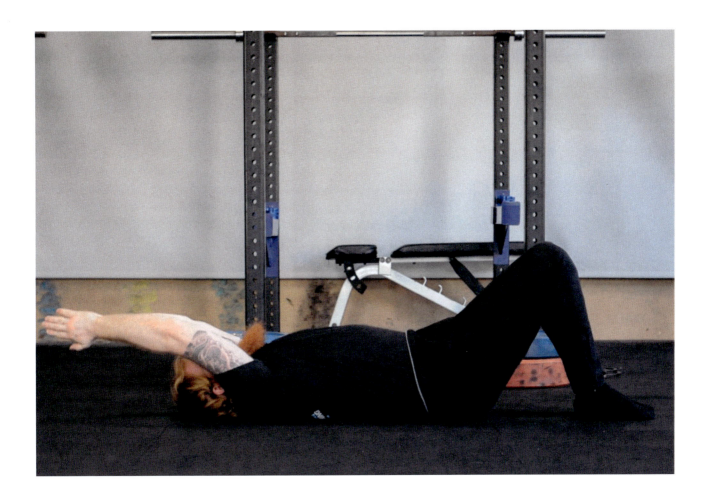

ASSESSING MOVEMENT

Assessing movement during a warm-up is one of the best ways to gather information about an individual's movement capabilities and specific areas such as balance and coordination.

During the first session with a client, I will usually start with a warm-up that allows me to see how they walk and run, squat, lunge, and perform basic exercises like a push-up. From there, the first gym-based session will involve a variant of a squat, single-leg, hinge, push, and pull exercise. Not only does this give me a lot of information in the first session, but it also limits DOMS and acts as a great intro to the gym. However, if someone needs a lot more work on the basics, a whole session might be dedicated to mastering squat and hinge mechanics.

Besides gathering information dynamically as we go, we can create movement assessments/screens, taking the individual through several assessments and grading them on their performance.

Movement assessments are often assessed on a 1-3 scale:

- 1 – Unable to attain the correct positioning/movement.

- 2 – Inconsistent positioning/movement.

- 3 – Maintains good positioning/movement throughout.

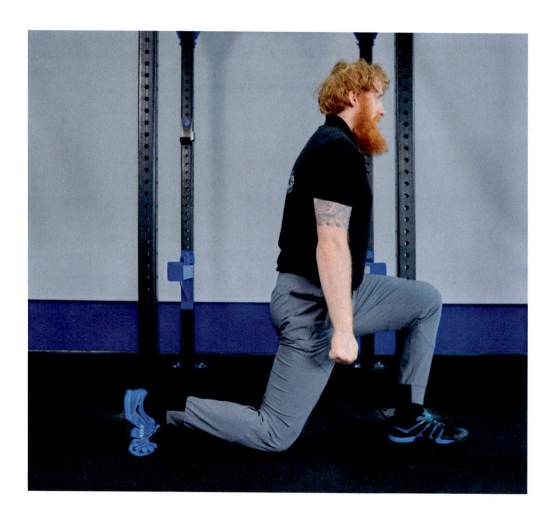

THE ATHLETIC ABILITY ASSESSMENT (AAA)

A study was carried out by Ian McKeown and published in the International Journal of Sports Physical Therapy. The study demonstrated the application of the Athletic Ability Assessment or AAA.

The AAA is an excellent example of a movement screen and only requires body weight or equipment usually accessible in gym environments. However, you could choose a selection of the below exercises.

Assessments: 9 Total

- **Prone Hold on Hands:** (High front plank) – 2 minutes.

- **Lateral Hold on Hands:** (High side plank) – 2 minutes – on each side.

- **Overhead Squat:** 10kg Olympic barbell x 5 reps.

- **Single-Leg Squat Off Box:** x 5 reps – on each side.

- **Walking Lunge:** 20kg Olympic barbell x 10 reps.

- **Single-Leg Forward Hop:** x 3 reps – on each side.

- **Lateral Bound:** x 3 reps – on each side

- **Push-Up:** Minimum of 20 reps for males / 12 reps for females.

- **Chin-Up:** Minimum of 10 reps for males / 4 reps for females.

Each exercise has 3 assessment points: Each exercise's maximum points are 9 (9 exercises = a total of 81).

Note: A "Chin-Up" refers to palms facing the individual, while a "Pull-Up" refers to palms facing away from the individual – even top athletes may find chin-ups extremely hard, especially if they have a heavier bodyweight.

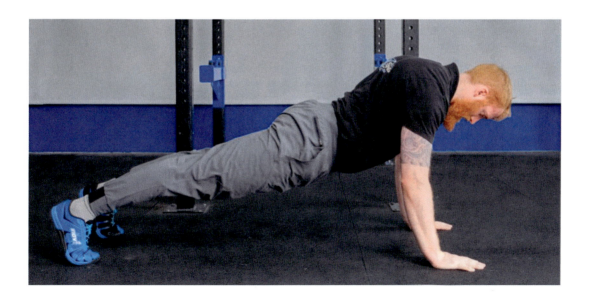

THE FUNCTIONAL MOVEMENT SCREEN (FMS)

The functional movement screen (FMS) is one of the most used tools to assess movement. However, it requires an FMS kit.

The FMS consists of 7 movement patterns, scored from 0-3 to create a total of 0-21 points: 0 is given if the individual has pain during any part of the movement.

- **Deep Squat:** Overhead squat with a dowel (included in the kit).

- **Hurdle Step:** With the dowel held across the individual's shoulders, the individual steps over a low hurdle and places their heel down before returning the foot to the starting position (the hurdle is created with the kit and set at the hight of the individual's tibial tuberosity – top of the shin, below the kneecap).

- **In-line Lunge:** Performed on the kit with a dowel held behind the individual's back with one arm behind the head and one arm behind the lower back, placing the dowel in-line with the spine.

- **Shoulder Mobility:** Back scratch test (one arm behind your lower back and reaching up, and the other arm over your shoulder and reaching down) measured with the dowel – the dowel has measurements on it.

- **Active Straight Leg Raise:** Lying on their back, the individual raises one leg while keeping both legs straight – the dowel is used to assess the leg position.

- **Trunk Stability Push-Up:** A push-up that is performed with the arms laid flat and the thumbs in line with the top of the forehead. This position results in the elbows being bent at 90 degrees.

- **Rotary Stability:** Bird Dog (pictured).

A score of <14 is used as the cut-off score. Individuals who score less than 14 points are thought to be at a greater risk of injury. However, the accuracy and applicability to specific sports and population groups are debated.

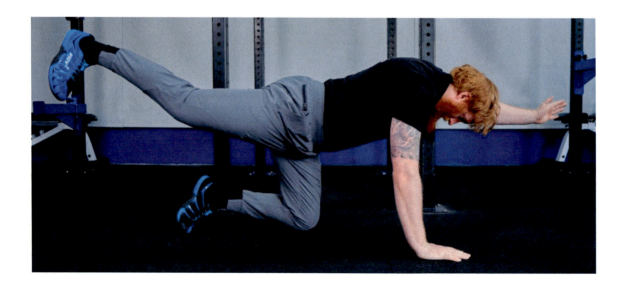

THE SCC MOVEMENT SCREEN (SCCMS)

Ultimately, you can add any movement that you believe to be applicable to a movement screening. However, just like any fitness test, we should ensure it provides us with useful data.

Here's an example of a standard movement screening used with clients and athletes at the SCC Academy:

- **Bodyweight Squat:** x 10 reps – movement basics and familiarity.

- **Overhead Squat:** x 3 reps with dowel (barbell can be used).

- **Bodyweight Walking Lunge:** x 10 reps – movement basics and familiarity.

- **Overhead Walking Lunge:** x 6 reps with dowel (barbell can be used).

- **Bodyweight Hip Hinge:** x 10 reps – movement basics and familiarity.

- **Dumbbell / Kettlebell Deadlift:** x 6 reps – 20kg for males / 16kg for females.

- **Vertical Countermovement Jump:** x 1 and x 3 (the x 3 are performed in quick succession).

- **Lateral Bounds:** x 4 reps with 1-second pause upon landing.

- **Slow Tempo Push-Ups:** x 6 reps for males / x 3 reps for females – tempo: 3131.

- **Barbell Overhead Press:** x 4 reps – 20kg for males / 10-15kg for females.

Scoring can be done using the 1-3 or 0-3 methods. However, we use a notes section for each, where technique faults, limitations, and compensations are recorded.

Examples:

Bodyweight Squat: "The athlete struggles to break parallel and experienced a high degree of knee valgus."

Bodyweight Hip Hinge: "The athlete was able to hip hinge while maintaining a neutral spine."

Vertical Countermovement Jump: "The athlete's stance was too wide and they became unstable upon landing – spent too much time on the ground in between successive jumps".

THE OVERHEAD SQUAT ASSESSMENT (OHSA)

Movement screens often involve several exercises performed one after the other. However, the overhead squat assessment (OHSA) is one of the quickest ways to gain an overall impression of an individual's functional status.

Note: Movement limitations and compensations should NOT be seen as a sure sign of injury risk, but as indicators to where improvements in overall performance can be made – making a more robust athlete!

The overhead squat assessment can be performed with or without a dowel:

- To perform the OHSA without a dowel, the individual adopts their squatting stance and raises their arms overhead while keeping their arms in-line with (covering) their ears.

- To perform the OHSA with a dowel, the individual adopts their squatting stance and holds the dowel in each hand at a width that when they place the dowel on the top of their head, their elbows are bent at 90 degrees. They then straighten their arms, keeping their arms in-line with (covering) their ears.

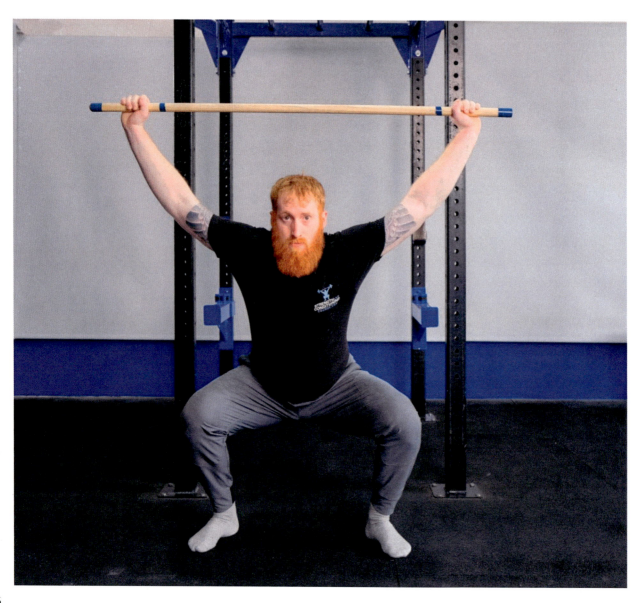

Once the individual reaches full depth, we look from a front and side view - the individual can reset between the front and side assessment to ensure they are not fatiguing at the bottom.

From the front view, we look at:

- Their feet – do their arches collapse, causing them to pronate/do their heels or toes raise (side view can be used)?

- Their knees – do they valgus?

- Their hips – is there a hip shift?

- Their shoulders – is one shoulder higher than the other?

Note: the hip area is often referred to as the lumbo-pelvic hip complex (LPHC), relating to the area around the hips, pelvis, and lower back.

From the side view, we look at:

- The LPHC – is there a prominent butt wink?

- The torso angle – is there excessive forward lean?

- The arm position – do the arms come forward of the ears?

- The head position – are they able to keep their head up?

From this assessment, we score the individual from 1-3 and make clear notes on areas for improvement.

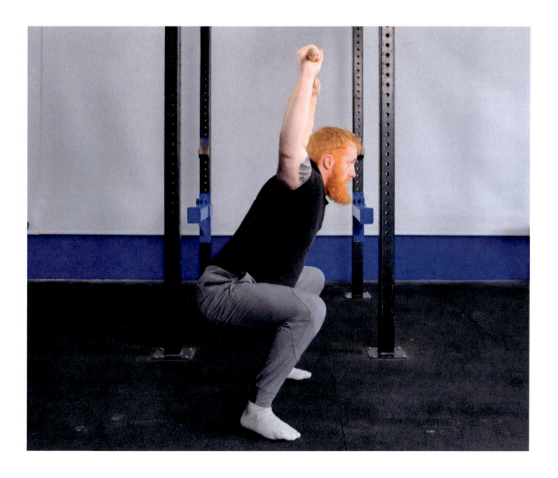

MOVEMENT IN ISOLATION

As discussed previously, there are 7 fundamental human movements that we use daily and develop with physical exercise.

For the most part, physical training should be based around working these complete movements, aka compound movements that work multiple joints and muscle groups. Compound movements give you more bang for your buck and usually result in greater adaptations (muscle mass and strength).

This being said, it is important to have an in-depth understanding of how each joint action is facilitated to create larger movements. This is important for building muscle and strength, keeping the tissues in good health, minimizing the risk of injuries, and rehabilitating specific issues.

In the following sections, we will work from the feet up to the neck and take an in-depth look at the muscles that surround the structures, the best way to release and stretch them, and the best way to work them through the movements they facilitate.

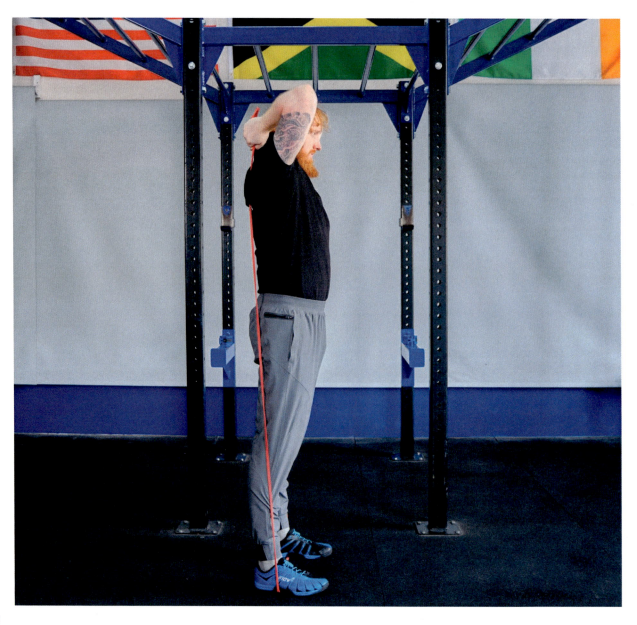

THE FEET

An entire book could be written about the importance of your feet. They are the foundations through which your entire weight is driven while standing, walking, and running or while squatting with a heavy weight on your back.

The breadth of issues various foot conditions can cause is expansive, and these issues can have knock-on effects throughout your entire body.

Many of the drills in this book can positively impact your feet, such as the many release techniques and stretches for your lower legs. However, in this section, I will be dealing with the feet directly.

When it comes to the health of your feet, try some barefoot walking. Warm them up by walking on your toes and heels, rotating your ankles, pointing your toes upwards towards your shin (dorsiflexion) and downwards towards the floor (plantarflexion). Move your toes around independently, separating your big toe from the other four and vice versa – all of this can be easily fitted in while at home.

Moreover, add in some basic release techniques and stretches that can help to maintain tissue health.

Note: Although footwear often gets a bad name from "barefoot advocates", there is clearly benefits to well cushioned trainers on a 26-mile run over concrete roads. However, it is good to allow the feet to do the work they were designed to do, which by nature would have been barefoot.

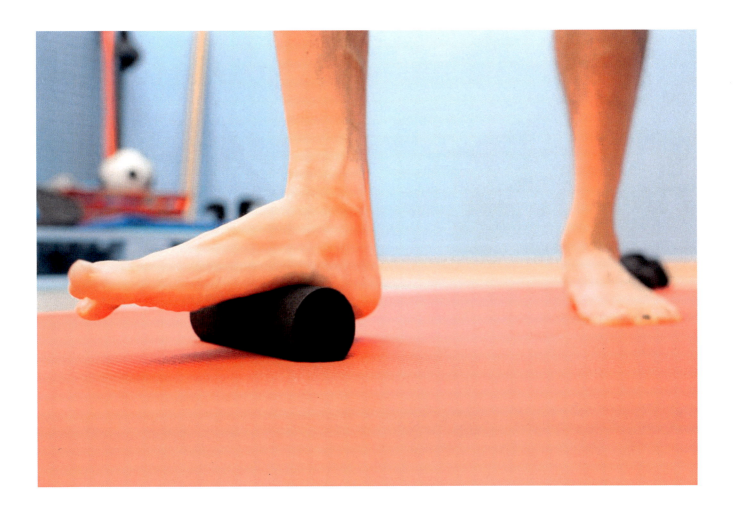

ROLLING THE FEET:

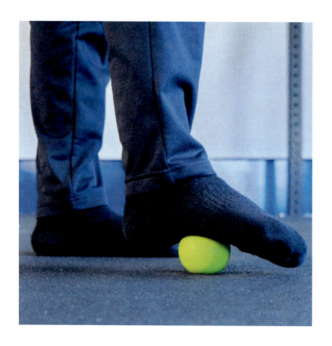

1. Stand up or sit on a bench or chair and place the massage ball or golf ball on the floor.
2. Place your foot on top of the ball and begin to roll the tissues on the sole of the foot.
3. Complete 1-3 sets of 30-60 seconds on each foot.

STANDING WALL STRETCH:

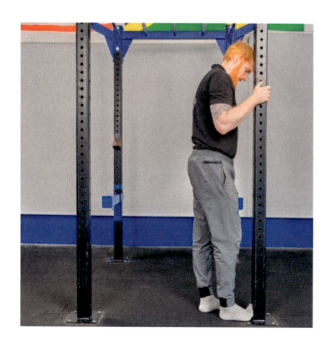

1. Stand up or sit on a bench or chair and place the massage ball or golf ball on the floor.
2. Place your right or left foot on top of the ball and begin to roll the tissues on the sole of the foot.
3. To increase the stretch, aim to keep your hips over your ankles.
4. Complete 1-3 sets of 30-60 seconds on each foot.

SEATED TOE AND ARCH STRETCH:

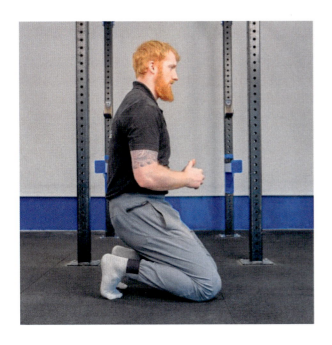

1. Tuck your toes under and kneel – your toes and knees should be supporting your weight.
2. Support your weight with your hands if needed.
3. Sit back onto your heels.
4. Hold for 30-60 seconds for a regular stretch or 2 minutes if the area is very tense.

STANDING TOP OF FOOT STRETCH:

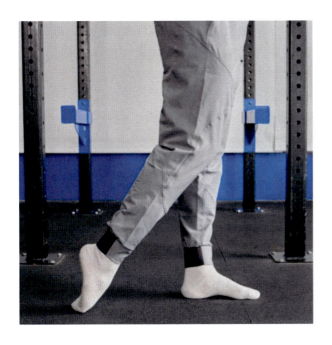

1. Stand with one foot flat on the ground.
2. Point your toes and place them down onto the floor.
3. The pointed foot can be placed slightly rearwards of the flat foot to achieve more of a tibialis anterior stretch.
4. Push down and forward slightly with the pointed foot.
5. Hold for 30-60 seconds for a regular stretch or 2 minutes if the area is very tense.

SEATED TOP OF FOOT STRETCH:

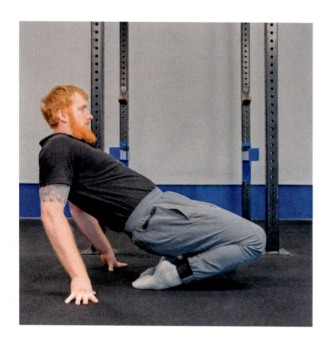

1. Kneel so that the tops of your feet are flat to the ground. Your toes should be facing rearwards.
2. Support your weight with your hands if needed.
3. To increase the stretch, sit back onto your heels, or raise your knees upwards by leaning back onto your hands.
4. Hold for 30-60 seconds for a regular stretch, or for 2 minutes if the area is very tense.

TOWEL CRUNCHES:

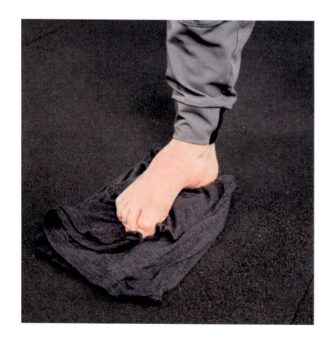

1. Spread a small towel on the floor.
2. Sit or stand at one end of the towel and place the toes of one foot onto the edge of the towel.
3. Raise your toes up, making sure your try to spread them apart.
4. Bring your toes down to the towel and use them to scrunch the towel up towards yourself.
5. Repeat this process until you have dragged the whole towel to your foot.
6. Once finished, spread the towel back out flat and complete successive sets on the same side, or change to the opposite foot.
7. Complete 3-5 sets on each side (depending on the length of the towel).

ANKLE ROLL-OUTS:

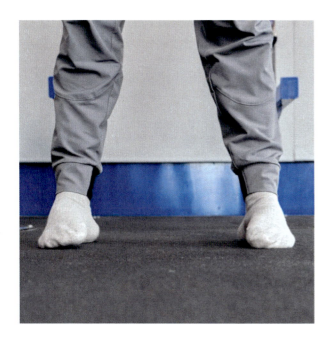

1. Stand up tall with good posture.
2. Push the outer side of your ankles outwards, while simultaneously gripping the floor with your big toe. You will feel the arch of your foot raising – use the muscles of your arch to drive upwards rather than just rolling over onto the outer side of your foot.
3. If performing this exercise with reps, hold the position for 1-2 seconds before coming back to your normal position – you can also push yourself into an exaggerated flat foot position to extend the range of motion.
4. If performing isometric holds, hold the position for 10-60 seconds, depending on the current strength of your arch
5. To progress the exercise, you can perform this drill on one leg, or add resistance by holding dumbbells or kettlebells.
6. Complete 10-15 reps on each side.

SINGLE-LEG BALANCE:

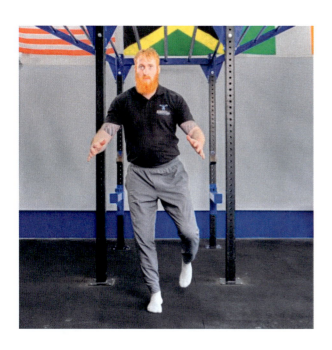

1. Stand on one leg.
2. Ensure your big toe, little toe and heel is down.
3. Hold the position for a set period or for as long as possible.
4. You can bend the knee and hip to increase the engagement of the leg muscles.

THE LOWER LEGS

Most of the muscles which control the movement of the feet are in your lower legs. Therefore, the lower legs play a huge role in how we move daily.

The lower legs also absorb a great deal of force when we walk, run and perform other ballistic activities. This is one of the reasons the bones of the lower leg (tibia and fibula) can often suffer fractures.

It is essential that we have strength in the lower leg muscles to help accommodate the stresses various activities place on them. However, many of the muscles in the lower legs become tense, causing pain, discomfort, and poor movement.

In this section, we look at:

- The Gastrocnemius and Soleus.

- The Peroneus Longus and Brevis.

- The Tibialis Anterior and Posterior.

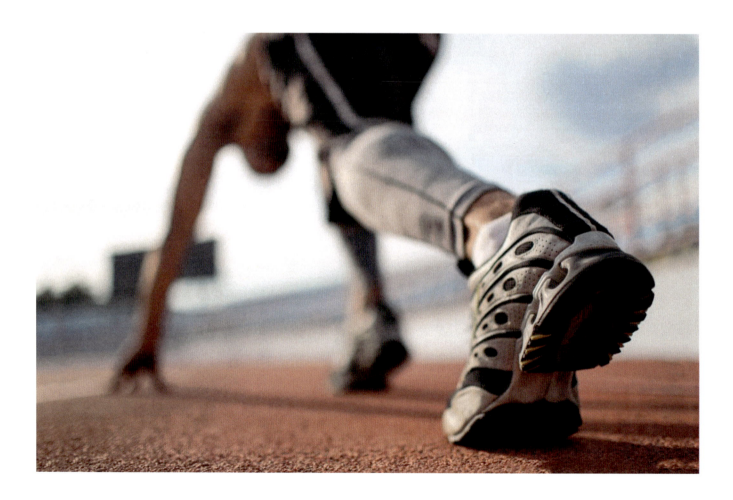

GASTROCNEMIUS

Origin	Posterior lower femur.
Insertion	Calcaneus via the calcaneal/Achilles' tendon.
Action	Plantarflexes the ankle and flexes the knee.
Antagonist	Tibialis anterior.
Innervation	Tibial nerve S1–S2.
Blood Supply	Sural arteries.
Daily Use	Walking, running (especially uphill), standing on your toes, climbing stairs, pedalling a bicycle.
Gym Use	Calf raises, squats, lunges, step-ups, leg press, single-leg balances, jumps.

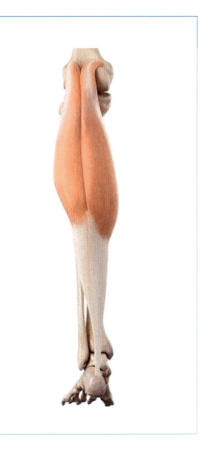

SOLEUS

Origin	Upper posterior tibia and fibula.
Insertion	Calcaneus via the calcaneal/Achilles' tendon.
Action	Plantarflexes the ankle.
Antagonist	Tibialis anterior.
Innervation	Tibial nerve S1-S2.
Blood Supply	Popliteal, posterior tibial, and peroneal (fibular) arteries.
Daily Use	Walking, running (especially uphill), standing on your toes, climbing stairs, pedalling a bicycle.
Gym Use	Calf raises, squats, lunges, step-ups, leg press, single-leg balances, jumps.

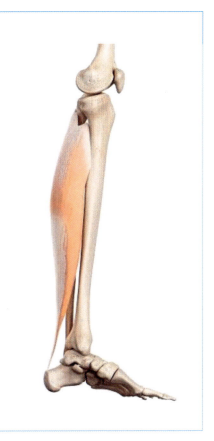

ROLLING THE CALVES:

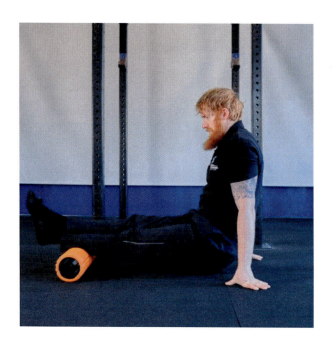

1. Sit on the floor and place a foam roller under your calves.
2. Both sides can be done at the same time if the roller is long enough but doing one at a time allows for more pressure to be placed through the calves.
3. If rolling your left leg, place your right foot over your left, then raise your body up with your hands.
4. Slowly roll up and down the muscles for 30-60 seconds. Do not roll over the back of the knee, as there are structures in your knee crease that don't respond well to rolling. Focus on the bulk of the muscle.
5. Complete 1-2 times on each side.

BARBELL ROLLING THE CALVES:

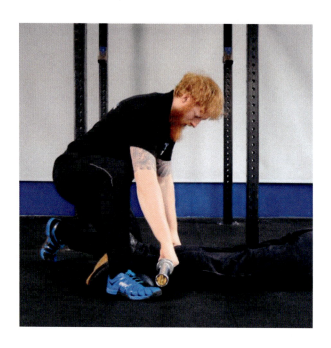

1. Instruct the client to lie on their front.
2. Place a barbell on the calves – use the appropriate load (discomfort not pain).
3. Slowly roll up and down the muscle for 30-60 seconds. Do not roll over the back of the knee, as there are structures in your knee crease that don't respond well to rolling. Focus on the bulk of the muscle.
4. Complete 1-2 times.

BARBELL ROLLING THE CALVES:

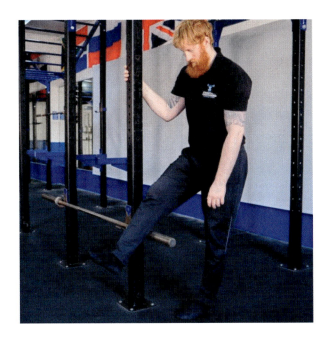

1. Set a barbell up on the rack at around knee height.
2. Stand behind the barbell so when you put your leg over the barbell, it pulls it back into the rack/J-cup (as pictured).
3. Place your leg over the sleeve to rest your calves on it.
4. Slowly roll up and down the muscle for 30-60 seconds.
5. Complete 1-2 times on each side.

HEEL DROP CALF STRETCH:

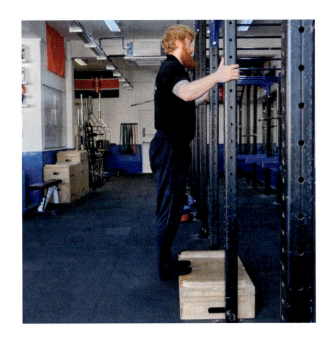

1. Stand with the balls of your feet on the edge of a step or platform.
2. Both legs can be stretched at once, or you can raise one leg up to apply more weight to the supporting leg and increase the stretch.
3. When stretching the gastroc, keep your knee(s) straight.
4. You can also change the angle at which your toes are pointing (inwards/forwards/outwards) to vary the stretch.
5. Bend your knee(s) slightly, and you will feel the stretch transition from your gastroc to your soleus (bending your knee(s) slacks the gastroc).
6. Repeat on both sides if stretching each leg independently.
7. Hold for 30-60 seconds, or 2 minutes if the musculature is very tense.
8. Complete 1-3 sets.

STANDING CALF STRETCH:

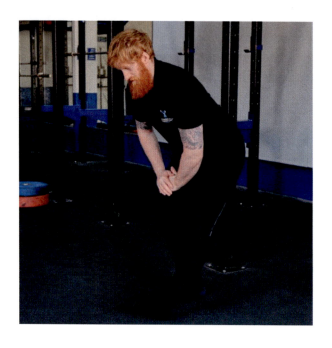

1. Stand in a hip-width stance and place one foot to the front with your heel down and your toes up.
2. Bend the rear leg and sit back with your glutes to increase the stretch.
3. Hold for 30-60 seconds, or 2 minutes if the musculature is very tense.
4. Complete 1-3 times on each side.

WALL CALF STRETCH:

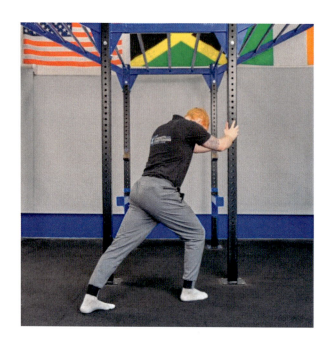

1. Take a long, split stance (lunge with a straight rear leg) and support yourself on a wall or post to your front.
2. While keeping the rear leg straight, drop your heel to the floor to stretch the calves.
3. Repeat on both sides.
4. Hold for 30-60 seconds, or 2 minutes if the musculature is very tense.
5. Complete 1-3 sets.

BAND ANKLE DORSIFLEXIONS:

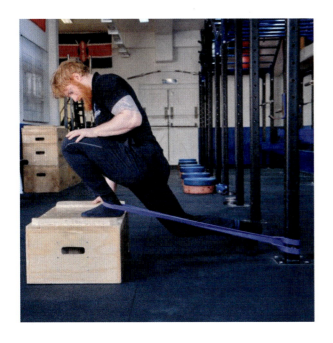

1. Attach a high-tension band around a solid structure.
2. Step into the band with one foot and place the band around the crease of your ankle.
3. Stride forward onto a low box with the banded leg to apply tension to the band – the aim is to pull the talus bone back.
4. Place both your hands onto your thigh and push your leg forward to dorsiflex the ankle – ensure you keep your heel down.
5. This position can be held for 30-60 seconds, or oscillations can be used, where you push into dorsiflexion then roll the knee outwards to bring yourself back to the starting position.
6. Repeat on both sides.
7. Complete 1-3 sets.

PARTNER CALF PNF:

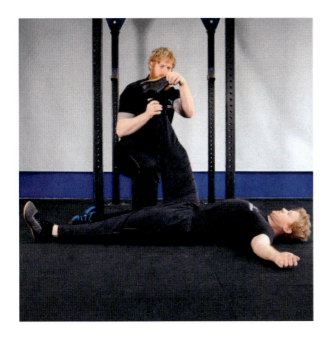

1. Have the client lie on their back.
2. Kneel and raise one of their legs to the barrier position for the back of the legs (hamstrings).
3. Place one hand just below their knee (on their thigh) and your other hand on the ball of their foot.
4. Push the ball of the foot down to create a calf stretch.
5. Hold the stretch for 10-15 seconds before releasing it slightly and instructing the client to push the ball of their foot into your hand.
6. Instruct the client to push with 50-60% intensity for 6-8 seconds.
7. Instruct the client to stop contracting and allow 1-2 seconds for the muscle to relax fully. During this time, instruct the client to take a deep breath in.
8. Instruct the client to exhale slowly, and as they do, push down on the ball of the foot to increase the stretch (reach a new barrier position) and hold for 10-15 seconds.
9. Repeat the previous steps 2-3 times and hold the final position for 20-30+ seconds.
10. Complete the stretch on both sides.

SOLO CALF PNF:

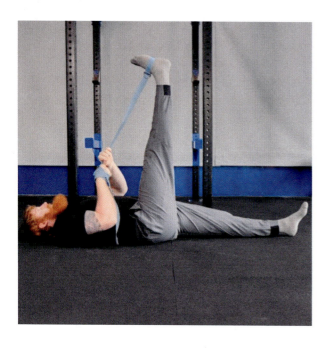

1. Stand on a step to create a heel drop.
2. Drop your heels to stretch your calves – straight knees to emphasize the gastrocnemius and bent knees to emphasize the soleus.
3. Hold the stretch for 10-15 seconds before going into a calf raise (straight or bent knees).
4. Hold the position for 6-8 seconds before dropping your heels to stretch the muscles and reach the new barrier position.
5. Repeat the previous steps 2-3 times and hold the final position for 20-30+ seconds.
6. This can be performed bilaterally or unilaterally.

GASTROCNEMIUS (CALF) RAISE:

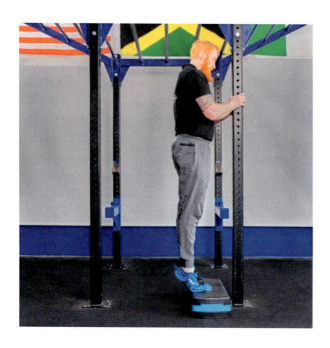

1. Step on a box or step with the balls of your feet. This exercise can also be performed without a heel drop (from the floor).
2. You can hold on to something with your hands for support.
3. Keep your knees straight to emphasize the work on the gastrocnemius.
4. Push the balls of your feet into the box to plantarflex your ankles – ensure you drive your big toes into the box.
5. This drill can be done bilaterally (both legs) or unilaterally (one leg at a time).
6. Complete 2-3 sets of 10-20 reps.

SOLEUS RAISE:

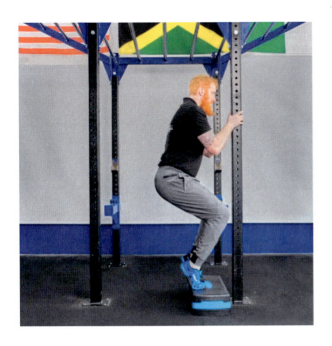

1. Step on a box or step with the balls of your feet. This exercise can also be performed without a heel drop (from the floor).
2. You can hold on to something with your hands for support.
3. Keep your knees bent to emphasize work on the soleus.
4. Push the balls of your feet into the box to plantarflex your ankles – ensure you drive your big toes into the box.
5. This drill can be done bilaterally (both legs) or unilaterally (one leg at a time).
6. Complete 2-3 sets of 10-20 reps.

SEATED SOLEUS RAISE:

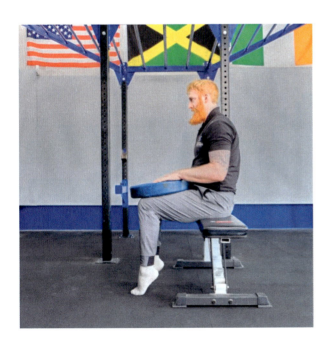

1. Sit on a bench.
2. Place a weight on your lap.
3. Push the balls of your feet into the floor (or a small block/step which creates a heel drop) to plantarflex your ankles – ensure you drive your big toes into the box.
4. This drill can be done bilaterally (both legs) or unilaterally (one leg at a time).
5. Complete 2-3 sets of 10-20 reps.

THE PERONEUS LONGUS AND BREVIS

PERONEUS LONGUS	
Origin	Upper lateral fibula.
Insertion	First metatarsal, medial cuneiform.
Action	Plantarflexes and everts the ankle.
Antagonist	Tibialis anterior.
Innervation	Superficial peroneal nerve L5-S1.
Blood Supply	Peroneal (fibular) artery.
Daily Use	Walking, running (especially on uneven surfaces – prevents inversion sprains).
Gym Use	Calf raises, single-leg balances, jumps.

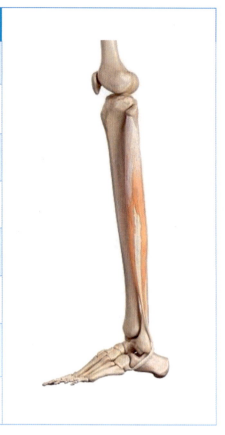

PERONEUS BREVIS	
Origin	Lower two-thirds of the lateral fibula.
Insertion	Fifth metatarsal.
Action	Plantarflexes and everts the ankle.
Antagonist	Tibialis anterior.
Innervation	Superficial peroneal nerve L5-S1.
Blood Supply	Personal (fibular) and anterior tibial arteries.
Daily Use	Walking, running (especially on uneven surfaces – prevents inversion sprains).
Gym Use	Calf raises, single-leg balances, jumps.

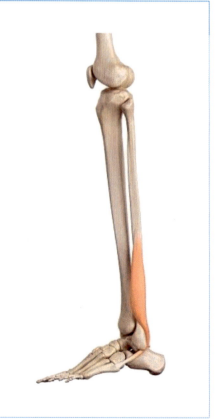

ROLLING THE PERONEUS:

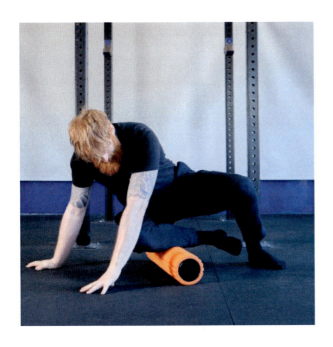

1. Place the foam roller onto the floor.
2. Place the outer side of one leg onto the foam roller.
3. While supporting yourself with your hands and your other foot, roll your peroneal group.
4. Slowly roll up and down the muscles for 30-60 seconds.
5. Complete 1-2 times on each side.

PERONEUS STRETCH:

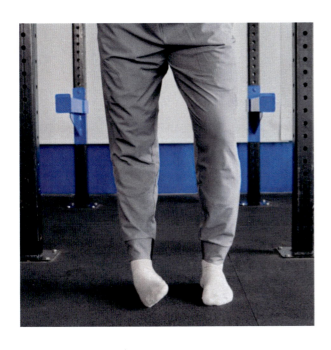

1. While standing, roll onto the outer side of one ankle and hold the position.
2. While seated, you can bring the soles of your feet together and allow your knees to drop outwards to feel the stretch on both sides.
3. Hold either position for 30-60 seconds or 2 minutes if the musculature is very tense.

BAND EVERSIONS:

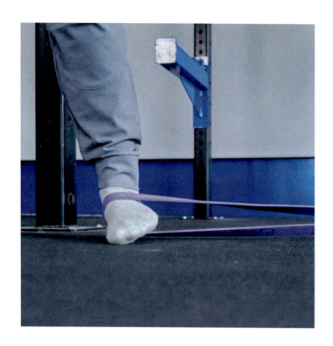

1. Attach a medium-high tension band to a solid structure.
2. Stand side-on to the band and place the closest foot to the band into it.
3. Step away from the band to apply tension to it.
4. Roll onto the inner side of the foot to evert the ankle before rolling back onto the outer side of the foot (inversion) to maximize the range of motion.
5. Complete 2-3 sets of 10 reps on each side.

EVERSION WALKING:

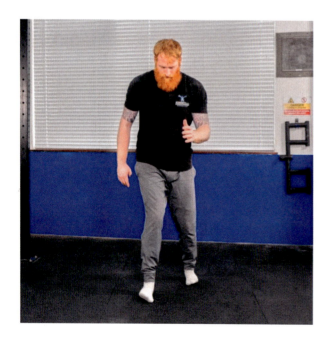

1. Push onto the inner side of the feet – this will bring the knees inwards (valgus).
2. In this position walk 10-20 strides.
3. Complete 2-3 sets of 10-20 strides.

THE TIBIALIS ANTERIOR

TIBIALIS ANTERIOR	
Origin	The upper half or two-thirds of the lateral surface of the tibia and the interosseous membrane.
Insertion	Medial cuneiform and the base of the first metatarsal.
Action	Dorsiflexes and inverts the ankle.
Antagonist	Tibialis posterior, gastrocnemius, soleus, plantaris, peroneus longus.
Innervation	Deep peroneal (fibular) nerve L4-L5.
Blood Supply	Anterior tibial artery.
Daily Use	Lifting foot while walking and running. Lifting foot while putting on your socks or shoes.
Gym Use	Band ankle dorsiflexions, single-leg balances.

ROLLING THE TIBILAIS ANTERIOR:

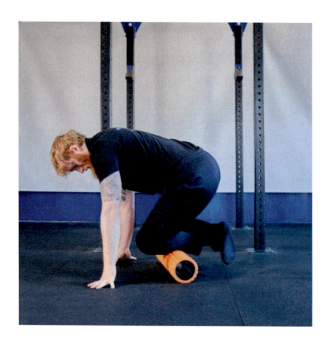

1. Place the foam roller onto the floor.
2. Place the front, outer side of one leg onto the foam roller. As if you are kneeling onto the roller with your shin (not your shin bone, but the muscles to the side).
3. Place your other leg over the back of the leg being rolled.
4. While supporting yourself with your hands, roll your tibialis anterior (you can also target your peroneal group from this position).
5. Slowly roll up and down the muscle for 30-60 seconds.
6. Complete 1-2 times on each side.

TIBIALIS ANTERIOR STRETCH:

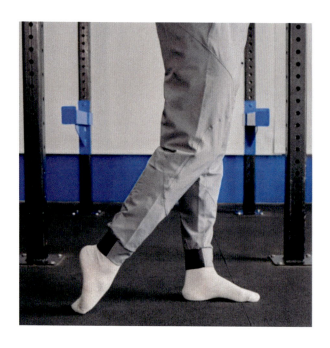

1. Stand with one foot flat on the ground.
2. Point your other foot with curled toes and place them down onto the floor.
3. The pointed foot should be placed slightly rearwards of the flat foot to achieve more of a tibialis anterior stretch.
4. Push down and forward slightly with the pointed foot.
5. Hold for 30-60 seconds for a regular stretch or 2 minutes if the area is very tense.

BAND DORSIFLEXIONS:

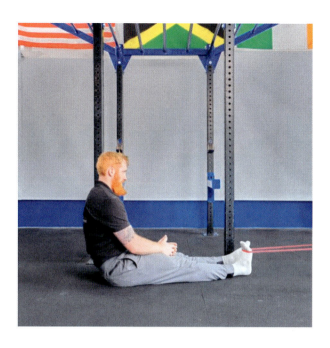

1. Attach a low-medium tension band to a solid structure.
2. Sit facing the band and wrap it around your foot.
3. Shuffle back to apply tension to the band.
4. Point your toes forward before dorsiflexing your ankle (toes towards your shins).
5. Complete 2-3 sets of 10-15 reps on each side.

HEEL WALKING:

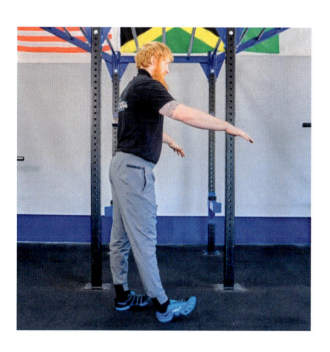

1. Come up onto your heels.
2. In this position walk 10-20 strides.
3. Complete 2-3 sets of 10-20 strides.

THE TIBIALIS POSTERIOR

TIBIALIS POSTERIOR	
Origin	Posterior surface of the tibia and fibula.
Insertion	Navicular and medial cuneiform bone.
Action	Inverts and plantarflexes the ankle.
Antagonist	Tibialis anterior, peroneus longus and brevis.
Innervation	Tibial nerve L4-L5.
Blood Supply	Posterior tibial artery.
Daily Use	Walking, running.
Gym Use	Calf raises, squats, lunges, step-ups, single-leg balances.

ROLLING THE TIBIALIS POSTERIOR:

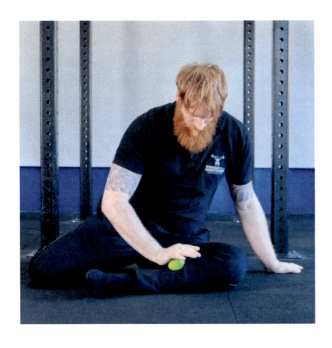

1. Sit on the floor and bring one heel in towards your groin so that the outer side of the lower leg is flat to the floor.
2. Place the massage ball just behind your shinbone and slowly roll it up and down the muscle, applying pressure with your hand.
3. Slowly roll up and down the muscle for 30-60 seconds.
4. Complete 1-2 times on each side.

TIBIALIS POSTERIOR STRETCH:

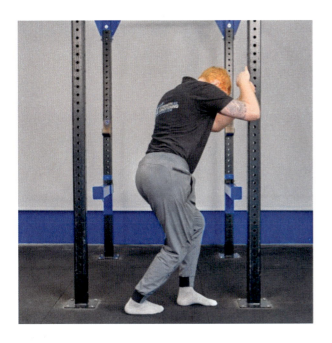

1. Stand in a split stance next to a wall. Your feet should be close together rather than the longer stride taken when stretching the calves.
2. Place your hands onto the wall for support.
3. Bend your knees, specifically the knee of your rear leg, to create a stretch.
4. To target the tibialis posterior specifically. Drop the same hip as the rear foot to the side.
5. Hold for 30-60 seconds, or 2 minutes if the musculature is very tense.
6. Complete 1-3 times on each side.

BAND PLANTARFLEXIONS AND EVERSIONS:

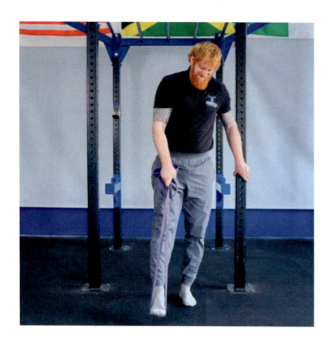

1. Tightly hold a medium to high tension band in your hands.
2. Place the ball of the foot into the band and flex your hip slightly to bring the foot off the ground while the leg is still straight.
3. If targeting the soleus, bend your knee. This can be assisted by pulling on the band.
4. Pull on the band to create tension and fully dorsiflex the ankle (toes towards the shin).
5. Push into the band with the ball of the foot to plantarflex the ankle (toes to the floor).
6. Push harder on the big toe side of the foot to evert the foot as it plantarflexes.
7. Perform 2-3 sets of 10-20 reps on each side.

TOE WALKING:

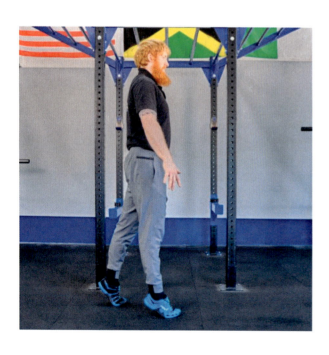

1. Come up onto your toes.
2. In this position walk 10-20 strides.
3. Complete 2-3 sets of 10-20 strides.

INVERSION WALKING:

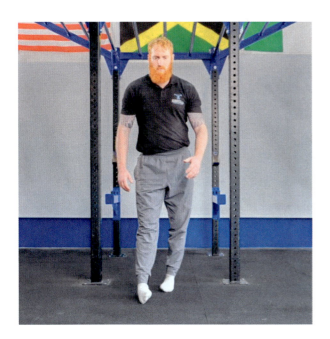

4. Come up onto the outer side of your feet.
5. In this position walk 10-20 strides.
6. Complete 2-3 sets of 10-20 strides.

THE UPPER LEGS

The muscles of the upper legs include some of the strongest muscles in your body. They are the driving force behind many of the movements you perform daily and in sport and physical training.

In this large section, the main muscle groups we look at are:

- The Quadriceps and Hip Flexors.

- The Adductors.

- The Hamstrings.

- The Gluteals.

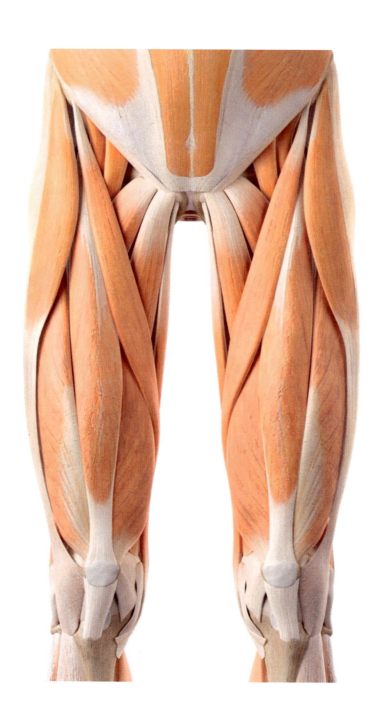

THE QUADRICEPS AND HIP FLEXORS

I have grouped the quadriceps and hip flexors together because they are easily released and stretched together. The TFL (another hip flexor) can also be easily rolled while doing the hip flexors and quads).

The quadriceps are made up of four muscles, the rectus femoris and the vastus muscles, vastus lateralis, vastus medialis, and vastus lateralis.

The rectus femoris (central quad muscle) crosses the hip joint and acts as a hip flexor (the sartorius muscle is another hip flexor).

The main hip flexor muscles are the psoas major and the iliacus, collectively known as the iliopsoas. The deep origin of the hip flexors means that you won't get a lot of release to the area. However, you can target some of the more superficial tissue that crosses your hip joint.

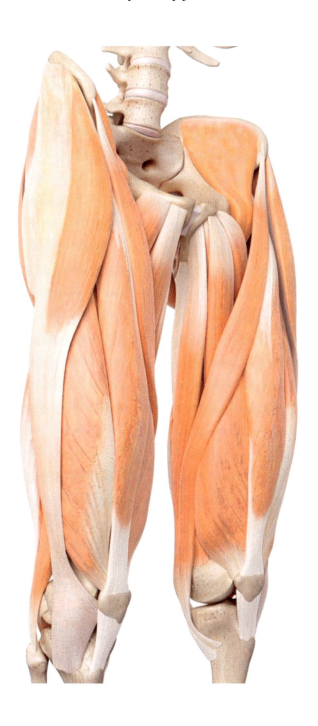

RECTUS FEMORIS

Origin	Anterior inferior iliac spine (AIIS).
Insertion	Patella via the patella tendon and tibial tuberosity via the patella tendon (actually a ligament).
Action	Extends the knee and flexes the hip.
Antagonist	Hamstrings.
Innervation	Femoral nerve L2-L4.
Blood Supply	Femoral, lateral femoral circumflex, superficial circumflex iliac arteries.
Daily Use	Standing up from sitting, walking, running, climbing stairs.
Gym Use	Squats, lunges, step-ups, leg press, leg extensions, single-leg balances, jumps.

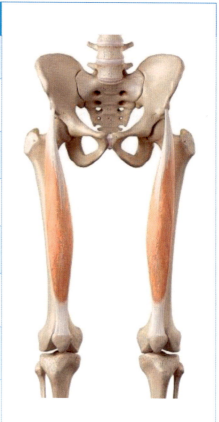

VASTUS LATERALIS

Origin	Greater trochanter.
Insertion	Patella via the patella tendon and tibial tuberosity via the patella tendon (actually a ligament).
Action	Extends the knee.
Antagonist	Hamstrings.
Innervation	Femoral nerve L2-L4.
Blood Supply	Lateral circumflex femoral and deep femoral arteries.
Daily Use	Standing up from sitting, walking, running, climbing stairs.
Gym Use	Squats, lunges, step-ups, leg press, leg extensions, single-leg balances, jumps.

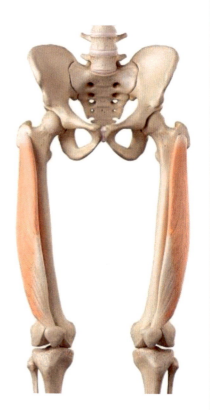

VASTUS MEDIALIS

Origin	Medial side of the femur.
Insertion	Patella via the patella tendon and tibial tuberosity via the patella tendon (actually a ligament).
Action	Extends the knee.
Antagonist	Hamstrings.
Innervation	Femoral nerve L2-L4.
Blood Supply	Femoral, deep femoral, descending genicular artery.
Daily Use	Standing up from sitting, walking, running, climbing stairs.
Gym Use	Squats, lunges, step-ups, leg press, leg extensions, single-leg balances, jumps.

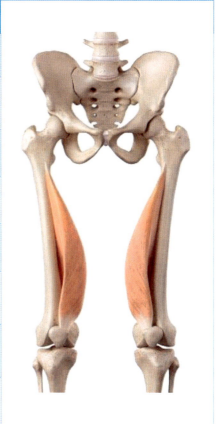

VASTUS INTERMEDIUS

Origin	Anterolateral femur.
Insertion	Patella via the patella tendon and tibial tuberosity via the patella tendon (actually a ligament).
Action	Extends the knee.
Antagonist	Hamstrings.
Innervation	Femoral nerve L2-L4.
Blood Supply	Deep femoral arteries.
Daily Use	Standing up from sitting, walking, running, climbing stairs.
Gym Use	Squats, lunges, step-ups, leg press, leg extensions, single-leg balances, jumps.

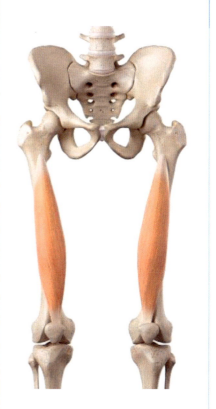

PSOAS MAJOR

Origin	Vertebral bodies of T12-L4, discs between T12-L4, transverse processes of L1-L5 vertebrae.
Insertion	Lesser trochanter of the femur.
Action	Flexes the hip.
Antagonist	Gluteus maximus.
Innervation	Anterior rami of spinal nerves L1-L3.
Blood Supply	Lumbar branch of the iliolumbar arteries.
Daily Use	Walking, running, sitting up (getting up out of bed).
Gym Use	Step-ups, lying or hanging leg raises, sit-ups, jack-knives, tuck jumps.

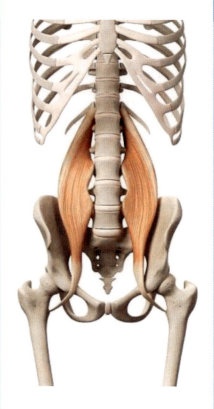

ILIACUS

Origin	Upper two-thirds of the iliac fossa.
Insertion	Lesser trochanter of the femur.
Action	Flexes and internally (medially) rotates the hip.
Antagonist	Gluteus maximus.
Innervation	Femoral nerve L1-L3.
Blood Supply	Iliolumbar, deep circumflex iliac, obturator, and femoral arteries.
Daily Use	Walking, running, sitting up (getting up out of bed).
Gym Use	Step-ups, lying or hanging leg raises, sit-ups, jack-knives, tuck jumps.

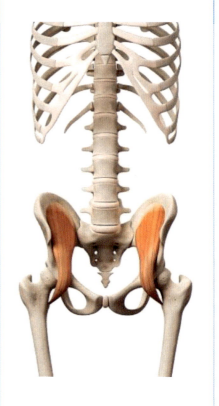

ROLLING THE QUADRICEPS AND HIP FLEXORS:

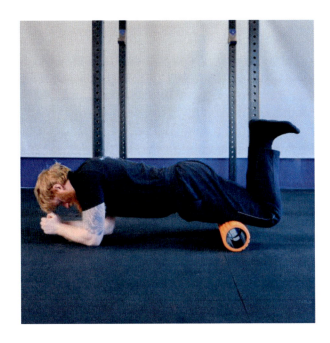

1. Place the foam roller or massage ball on the floor.
2. To roll the hip flexors. Lie onto the roller at the crease of your hip on one side – practice caution when placing a massage ball into the crease of the hip or groin to not overly stress the area.
3. To roll the quadriceps, roll up and down the entire length of the thigh – one or both legs can be rolled at a time, and you can rotate your leg to target the inner or outer side of the thighs.
4. Slowly roll up and down the muscle mass for 30-60 seconds.
5. Complete 1-2 sets on each side.

BARBELL ROLLING THE QUADRICEPS:

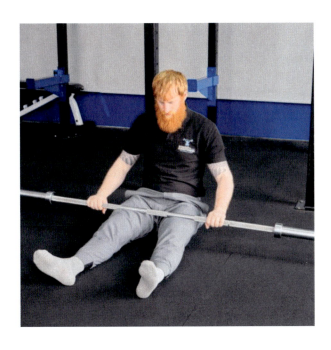

1. Sit on the floor with your legs straight – you can sit with your back against a wall for support.
2. Place a barbell on your quadriceps – use the appropriate load (discomfort not pain).
3. Slowly roll up and down the muscle for 30-60 seconds.
4. Complete 1-2 times.

HALF-KNEELING QUADRICEPS AND HIP FLEXOR STRETCH:

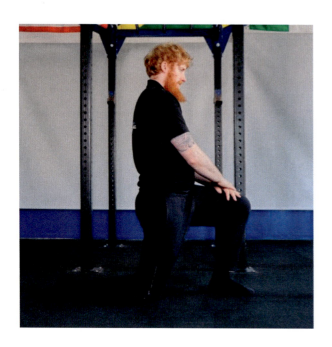

1. Adopt a half-kneeling position.
2. If stretching your right side, squeeze your glutes, focusing on the right side, and drive your right hip forward into hyperextension to facilitate the stretch. Your pelvis should remain neutral throughout.
3. Raising the same arm to the hip flexor you are stretching and reaching over the opposite shoulder increases the stretch through the hip flexors quad and abdominals.
4. Hold for 30-60 seconds, or 2 minutes if the musculature is very tense.
5. Complete 1-3 times on each side.

HALF-KNEELING STRETCH WITH POSTERIOR BAND DISTRACTION:

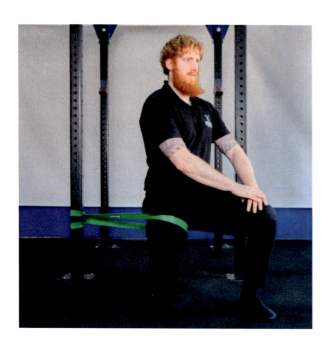

1. Attach a high-tension band around a solid structure.
2. Step into the band and loop it around the top of your leg (pull it right into your groin).
3. Stride forward with your opposite leg and bring your rear knee down to apply tension to the band.
4. Push forward with the rear hip to apply the stretch to your hip flexors.
5. Hold for 30-60 seconds, or 2 minutes if the musculature is very tense.
6. Complete 1-3 times on each side.

COUCH QUADRICEPS AND HIP FLEXOR STRETCH:

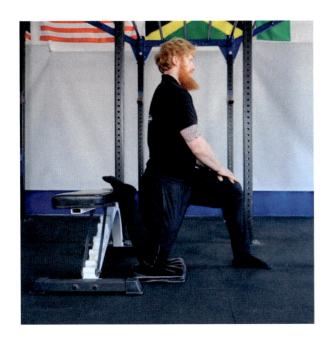

1. Place your right leg against a wall or the top of your foot onto a raised platform that is just below knee height.
2. This places you in a half-kneeling position with your left foot flat on the floor to the front.
3. Squeeze your glutes, specifically the right side, and drive your right hip forward into hyper-extension to facilitate the stretch. Your pelvis should remain neutral.
4. Raising the arm on the side of the stretch and reaching over the opposite shoulder increases the stretch.
5. Hold for 30-60 seconds, or 2 minutes if the musculature is very tense.
6. Complete 1-3 times on each side.

STANDING QUADRICEPS STRETCH:

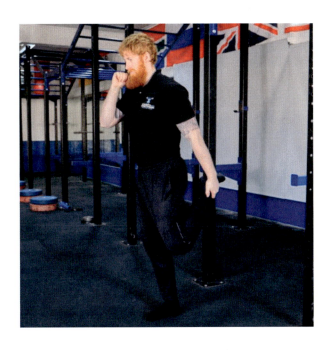

1. From a standing position, grab the top of one foot.
2. Maintain a soft knee position with the supporting leg.
3. Pull the foot up towards your glutes.
4. Keep your knees close together, which ensures you maintain a full stretch down the length of your quads.
5. Squeeze your glutes, focusing on the side you are stretching, and drive the hip forward into hyperextension to facilitate the stretch. Your pelvis should remain neutral throughout.
6. Hold for 30-60 seconds, or 2 minutes if the musculature is very tense.
7. Complete 1-3 times on each side.

LYING QUADRICEPS STRETCH:

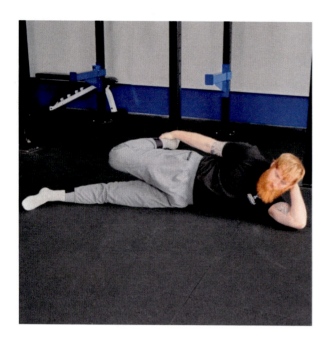

1. While lying on your side, grab the top of your foot.
2. Pull your foot up towards your glutes, keep your knees close together. This ensures you maintain a full stretch down the length of your quads.
3. Squeeze your glutes, focusing on the side you are stretching, and drive the hip forward into hyperextension to facilitate the stretch. Your pelvis should remain neutral throughout.
4. Hold for 30-60 seconds, or 2 minutes if the musculature is very tense.
5. Complete 1-3 times on each side.

KNEELING QUADRICEPS STRETCH:

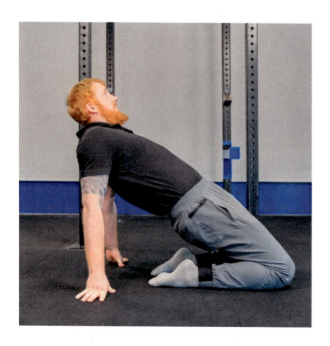

1. Kneel on the floor.
2. Lean back and place your hands on the floor to the rear.
3. Squeeze your glutes to raise your hips up to apply the stretch to your quads.
4. Hold for 30-60 seconds, or 2 minutes if the musculature is very tense.
5. Complete 1-3 times on each side.

PARTNER QUADRICEPS AND HIP FLEXOR PNF:

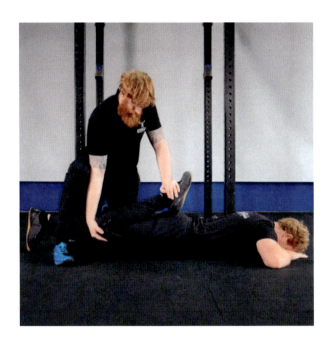

1. Instruct the client to lie on their front.
2. Bend one of their legs to bring their heel towards their glutes.
3. Hold the foot down with one hand and place your other hand on the bottom of the bent quad to lift it up to increase the stretch.
4. Hold the stretch for 10-15 seconds before releasing it slightly.
5. Instruct the client to push their leg toward the floor to engage their hip flexors and/or their foot against your hands to engage your quads – 50-60% intensity for 6-8 seconds.
6. Instruct them to stop contracting and to take a deep breath in and allow 1-2 seconds for the muscle to relax fully.
7. Instruct them to exhale slowly and as they do, push their foot into their glute and raise their leg to increase the stretch and hold for 10-15 seconds.
8. Repeat the previous steps 2-3 times and hold the final position for 20-30+ seconds.
9. Complete the stretch on both sides.

SOLO QUADRICEPS AND HIP FLEXOR PNF:

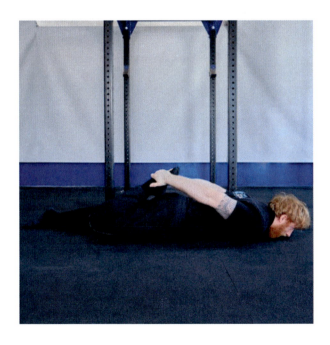

1. Lie on your front.
2. Bend your knee, bring your arms behind your back, and grab the foot of the bent leg.
3. Pull the leg up to stretch hip flexors and quadriceps.
4. Hold the stretch for 10-15 seconds before releasing it slightly.
5. Push your leg toward the floor to engage your hip flexors and/or your foot against your hands to engage your quads – 50-60% intensity for 6-8 seconds.
6. Stop contracting and allow 1-2 seconds for the muscle to relax fully, and take a deep breath in.
7. Exhale slowly and pull on the foot to increase the stretch and hold for 10-15 seconds.
8. Repeat the previous steps 2-3 times and hold the final position for 20-30+ seconds.
9. Complete the stretch on both sides.

SOLO QUADRICEPS AND HIP FLEXOR PNF WITH STRAP:

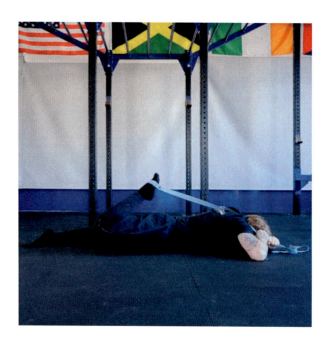

1. Loop a strap or resistance band around your foot.
2. Hold the strap in your hands and lie on your front.
3. Pull on the strap to bring your foot towards your glutes and raise the bent leg off the floor.
4. Pull the leg up to stretch hip flexors and quadriceps.
5. Hold the stretch for 10-15 seconds before releasing it slightly.
6. Push your leg toward the floor to engage your hip flexors and/or your foot against the strap to engage your quads – 50-60% intensity for 6-8 seconds.
7. Stop contracting and allow 1-2 seconds for the muscle to relax fully, and take a deep breath in.
8. Exhale slowly and pull on the foot to increase the stretch and hold for 10-15 seconds.
9. Repeat the previous steps 2-3 times and hold the final position for 20-30+ seconds.
10. Complete the stretch on both sides.

TERMINAL KNEE EXTENSIONS:

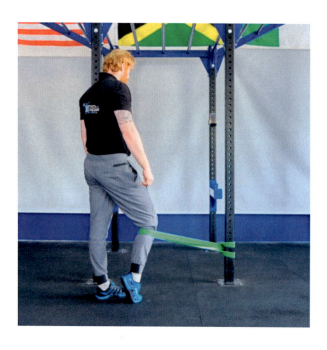

1. Place a medium to high tension band around something solid at knee height.
2. Step into the band with one leg and place the band around the back of the knee (in the crease).
3. Step back to apply tension to the band.
4. With the leg that is attached to the band, slowly roll forward onto the ball of the foot to bend your knee.
5. Slowly bring your foot back down onto your heel and lock your knee fully, ensuring you don't place unnecessary stress on the joint by forcing it into a hyperextension.
6. Complete 3-4 sets of 15-20 reps on each side.

BAND QUADRICEPS EXTENSIONS:

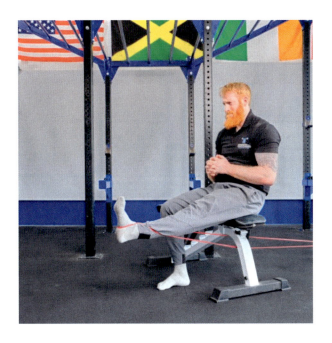

1. Attach a low-tension band to a solid structure.
2. Sit on a bench facing away from the band.
3. Grab the band and loop it around your foot (bottom of your shin) – you can loop it around 2-3 times.
4. Engage your quadriceps to extend the knee.
5. Squeeze the quadriceps hard at the top of the movement.
6. Compete 2-3 sets of 10-15 reps.

SPANISH SQUATS:

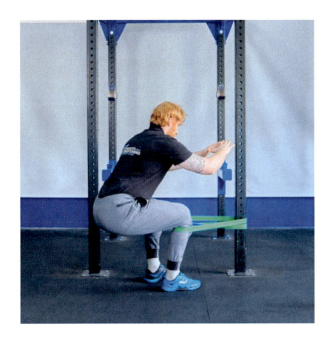

1. Attach 1-2 medium to high tension resistance bands around a solid structure.
2. Step into the band(s) so that they are placed at the top of the calves.
3. Walk back to apply tension to the bands – the bands will support you as you sit back but will not save you from falling.
4. Sit back into a parallel squat with your shins vertical – the bands allow for this.
5. Hold this position for 30-40 seconds.
6. After the isometric hold, you can perform 5-10 squats to really get the quads firing (keep the shins vertical).
7. Complete 2-3 sets of 30-40 second holds and include 5-10 squats at the end of the hold.

PSOAS MARCHES:

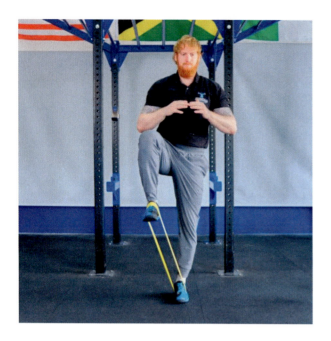

1. Sit on the floor and place the band around the centre of your feet.
2. Lie back, so your head is flat on the floor.
3. Bend your knees and raise your feet up, bringing your legs right back towards your torso.
4. Slowly extend your left leg while ensuring your right leg remains in a fully flexed position.
5. Slowly return your left leg back to a flexed position and proceed to extend your right leg.
6. If performing the drill standing up, place the band around the centre of your feet and stand up tall with good posture or lean against a post/wall.
7. Flex one hip through a full ROM before bringing it back to the floor and flexing the other hip.
8. Complete 2-3 sets of 10-20 reps on each side.

STANDING HIP FLEXOR HOLDS:

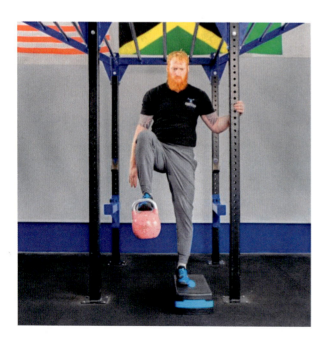

1. Stand on a low step or box with one leg.
2. Hook your foot under the handle (horn) of a kettlebell.
3. Flex your hip to raise your knee up as high as possible.
4. Hold the position for 20-40 seconds.
5. Complete 2-3 sets of 20-40 second holds.

THE ADDUCTORS

The adductors are a large group of muscles on your inner thigh that are responsible for bringing your legs back towards your body from the side. While running, they draw your legs together to control swinging and help to stabilize your stride.

The main adductors are:

- Adductor Magnus.

- Adductor Longus.

- Adductor Brevis.

- Pectineus.

- Gracilis.

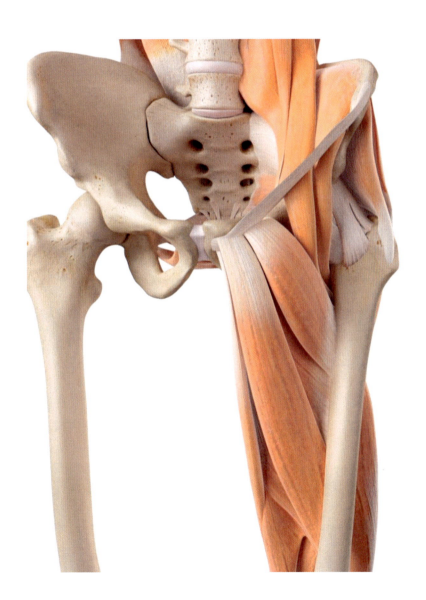

ADDUCTOR MAGNUS

Origin	Pubis and tuberosity of the ischium.
Insertion	Linea aspera (posterior surface of the femur) and the adductor tubercle of the femur.
Action	Adducts the hip.
Antagonist	Gluteus medius.
Innervation	Posterior branch of the obturator nerve L2-L4. Tibial division of sciatic nerve L4.
Blood Supply	Deep femoral artery.
Daily Use	Walking, running, wood chopping, horse riding, ice skating.
Gym Use	Squats, lunges, hip adductions, single-leg balances, jumps.

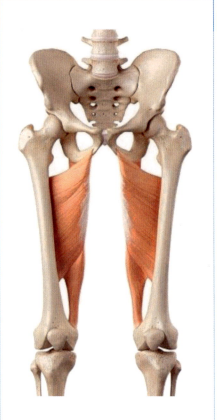

ADDUCTOR LONGUS

Origin	Pubic body just below pubic crest.
Insertion	Middle third of the linea aspera (posterior surface of the femur).
Action	Adducts and flexes the hip.
Antagonist	Gluteus medius.
Innervation	Obturator nerve L2-L4.
Blood Supply	Profunda femoris and obturator artery.
Daily Use	Walking, running, wood chopping, horse riding, ice skating.
Gym Use	Squats, lunges, hip adductions, single-leg balances, jumps.

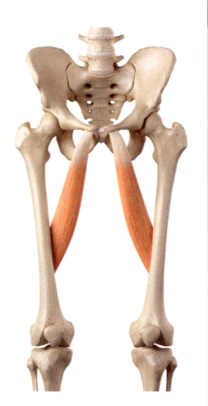

ADDUCTOR BREVIS	
Origin	Anterior surface of the inferior ramus and body of the pubis.
Insertion	The lesser trochanter and linea aspera (posterior surface of the femur).
Action	Adducts the hip.
Antagonist	Gluteus medius.
Innervation	Obturator nerve L2-L4.
Blood Supply	Arteria profunda femoris.
Daily Use	Walking, running, wood chopping, horse riding, ice skating.
Gym Use	Squats, lunges, hip adductions, single-leg balances, jumps.

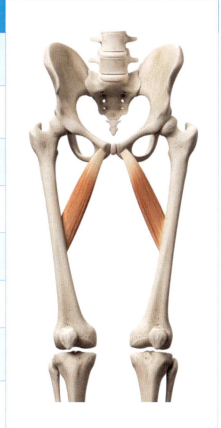

PECTINEUS	
Origin	Anterior, superior pubis.
Insertion	Posterior, upper femur.
Action	Adducts, flexes and internally (medially) rotates the hip.
Antagonist	Gluteus medius.
Innervation	Femoral nerve and obturator nerve L2-L3.
Blood Supply	Medial femoral circumflex and obturator arteries.
Daily Use	Walking, running, wood chopping, horse riding, ice skating.
Gym Use	Squats, lunges, hip adductions, single-leg balances, jumps.

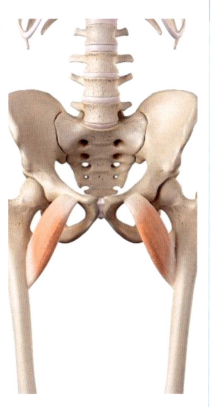

GRACILIS	
Origin	Anterior, inferior pubis.
Insertion	Medial, upper tibia – Pes Anserinus.
Action	Adducts and internally (medially) rotates the hips and flexes the knee.
Antagonist	Gluteus medius.
Innervation	Obturator nerve L2-L2.
Blood Supply	Deep femoral artery.
Daily Use	Walking, running, wood chopping, horse riding, ice skating.
Gym Use	Squats, lunges, hip adductions, single-leg balances, jumps.

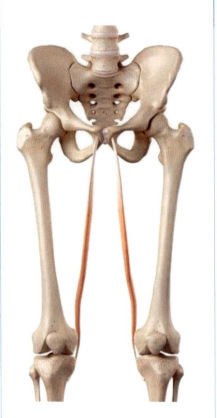

ROLLING THE ADDUCTORS:

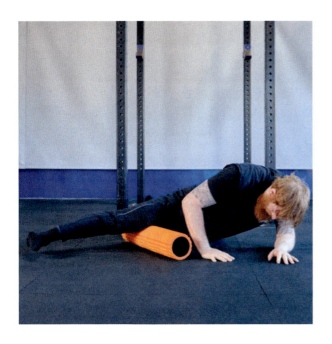

1. Lie face down on the floor with the roller to your side, at your hips.
2. Raise the leg you are rolling out to the side and place your inner thigh on the roller.
3. If you can't raise your leg to the roller, simply lower it down, ensuring the roller ends up perpendicular to your leg.
4. Use your hands/forearms to raise your body up to apply more pressure onto the foam roller.
5. Slowly roll up and down the muscle mass for 30-60 seconds.
6. Complete 1-2 times on each side.

BARBELL ROLLING THE ADDUCTORS:

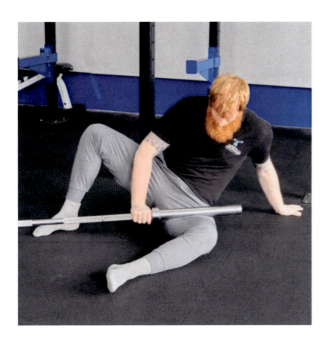

1. Sit on the floor and place one leg out to the side.
2. Place the sleeve of the barbell onto your inner thigh.
3. Slowly roll up and down the muscle for 30-60 seconds.
4. Complete 1-2 times on each side.

BUTTERFLY ADDUCTOR STRETCH:

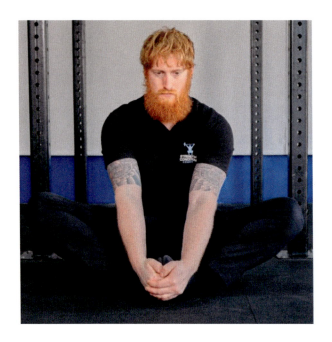

1. Sit on the floor and place the soles of your feet together.
2. Pull your heels in towards your groin.
3. Hold onto the balls of your feet.
4. Lean forward with your torso, keeping your spine straight, and push your knees towards the floor.
5. Hold for 30-60 seconds, or 2 minutes if the musculature is very tense.
6. Complete 1-3 times.

FROG ADDUCTOR STRETCH:

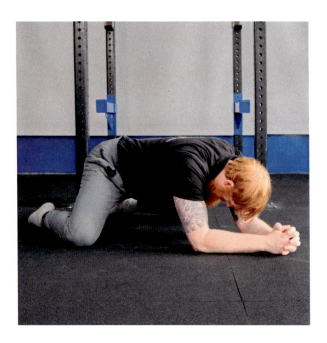

1. Get down into a quadruped position.
2. Spread your legs so your knees are as far apart as possible.
3. Sit back with your hips/glutes to apply a stretch to your inner thighs.
4. As you sit back with your hips, you can come down onto your forearms.
5. Hold for 30-60 seconds, or 2 minutes if the musculature is very tense – you can also create a dynamic stretch by moving forward and back (oscillatory stretch).
6. Complete 1-3 times.

FROG STRETCH WITH LATERAL BAND DISTRACTIONS:

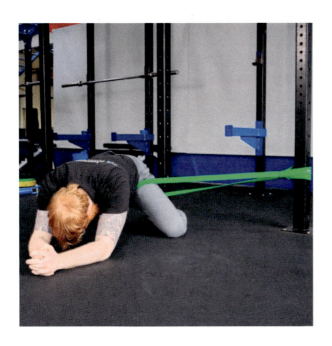

1. Attach a high-tension band around a solid structure.
2. Step into the band and loop it around the top of your leg (pull it into your groin).
3. Sidestep away from the band attachment point to apply tension to the band.
4. Drop down into the frog stretch position.
5. Hold for 30-60 seconds, or 2 minutes if the musculature is very tense.
6. Complete 1-3 times on each side.

LYING ADDUCTOR STRETCH:

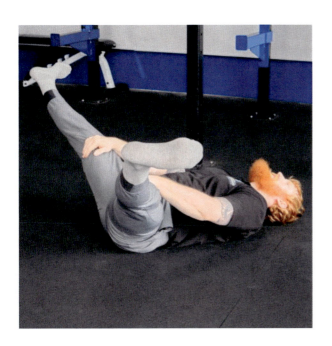

1. Lie on your back and raise your legs up while keeping your knees straight.
2. Open your legs (drop your legs to either side) and push on your inner thighs to increase the stretch.
3. Hold for 30-60 seconds, or 2 minutes if the musculature is very tense.
4. Complete 1-3 times.

DEEP SQUAT ADDUCTOR STRETCH

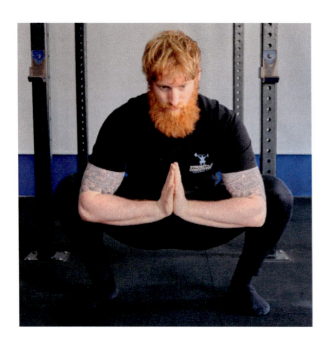

1. Stand with your feet shoulder-width apart. Toes can be angled out slightly.
2. Squat down into the deepest squat you can achieve. Try to maintain a neutral spine with a proud chest.
3. Some lumbar flexion (where your lower back rounds slightly as your pelvis tilts underneath) in a deep squat is normal. Just ensure it is not excessive or putting stress on your lower back.
4. Place your hands into a prayer position and use your elbows to push your knees outwards.
5. Hold for 30-60 seconds, or 2 minutes if the musculature is very tense.
6. Complete 1-3 times.

90/90 STRETCH:

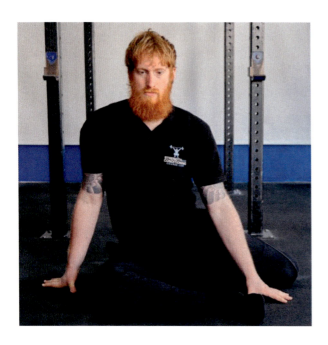

1. Sit on the floor and bring one leg to the front and one leg to rear with your knees bent at 90 degrees.
2. Your front leg will be rested on the outer side of the leg and the rear leg will be rested on the inner side of the leg – the hip of the front leg is externally rotated, and the hip of the rear leg is internally rotated.
3. Try to keep your torso upright – you will find you lean to the side of your front leg if there is tension around the hips and lower spine.
4. This stretch can be performed dynamically, fluidly transitioning from one side to the other without having your hands on the floor.
5. Hold for 30-60 seconds, or 2 minutes if the musculature is very tense.
6. Complete 1-3 times on each side.

PARTNER ADDUCTOR PNF:

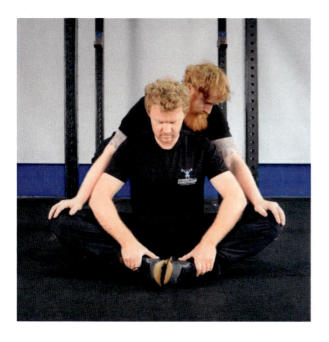

1. Have the client sit in the butterfly stretch position – legs bent with the soles of their feet together.
2. Kneel behind the client and place your hands on their inner thighs (close to their knees).
3. Push down on their thighs to create a stretch on their inner thighs.
4. Hold the stretch for 10-15 seconds before releasing it slightly and instructing the client to push their inner thighs into your hands.
5. Instruct the client to push with 50-60% intensity for 6-8 seconds.
6. Instruct the client to stop contracting and allow 1-2 seconds for the muscles to relax fully. During this time, instruct the client to take a deep breath in.
7. Instruct the client to exhale slowly, and as they do, push down on their inner thighs to increase the stretch, and hold for 10-15 seconds.
8. Repeat the previous steps 2-3 times and hold the final position for 20-30+ seconds.

SOLO ADDUCTOR PNF:

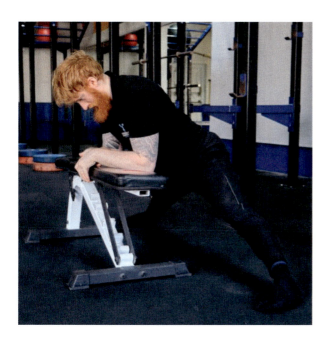

1. Depending on how low you can go, support yourself with your hands or forearms on a bench, box, or sofa, etc.
2. Spread your legs into a box (side/center) split position. A front split position can also be used, which places more stretch onto the front leg's hamstrings.
3. Hold the stretch for 10-15 seconds before releasing it slightly.
4. Engage the muscles you are stretching by contracting the muscles as if you are going to pull yourself up out of the split position using your legs alone – 50-60% intensity for 6-8 seconds.
5. Stop contracting and allow 1-2 seconds for the muscles to relax fully, and take a deep breath in.
6. Exhale slowly and lower yourself down into a deep split position to increase the stretch and hold for 10-15 seconds.
7. Repeat the previous steps 2-3 times and hold the final position for 20-30+ seconds.
8. Complete the stretch on both sides if performing front splits.

LYING MEDICINE BALL SQUEEZE:

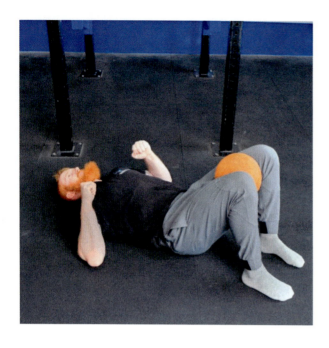

1. Lie on your back.
2. Bend your knees and place your feet flat on the floor.
3. Open your legs (knees fall out to the sides) and place a medicine ball between your legs (close to your knees).
4. Squeeze the ball for 15-40 seconds.
5. Complete 2-3 sets of 15-40 seconds.

STANDING BAND ADDUCTIONS:

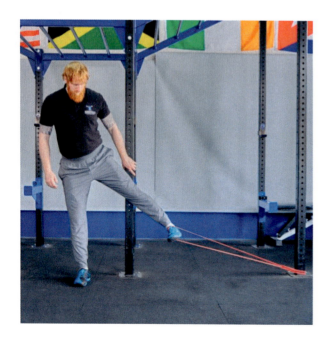

1. Attach a low-tension band to the bottom of a post.
2. Stand side on to the band attachment point and loop the band around the foot closest to the post.
3. Step away from the post to apply tension to the band while the leg is abducted (to the side and off the floor).
4. This drill can be performed without holding onto something for support, which doubles as a stability drill. Or you can hold onto something and really concentrate on the adducting leg – it creates quite an intense burn.
5. Adduct the leg (pull the leg into the supporting leg).
6. Complete 2-3 sets of 10-20 reps on each side.

THE HAMSTRINGS

The hamstrings work to extend the hips and flex the knees. This means they work incredibly hard when we run. Therefore, rolling and stretching the hamstrings can help to keep them in good health.

When it comes to hamstring tightness, it is important to consider how other muscles are having an impact, specifically those that also attach to the pelvis and perform the same actions. If surrounding muscles are not pulling their weight, others might have to compensate – working your glutes, calves, and abdominals can help.

The hamstrings are made up of:

- Biceps Femoris.

- Semimembranosus.

- Semitendinosus.

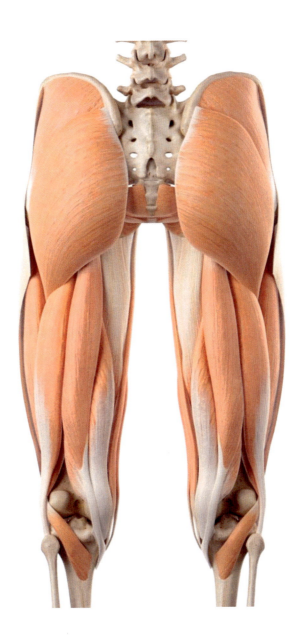

BICEPS FEMORIS

Origin	Long head: Ischial tuberosity / Short head: Posterior surface of the femur.
Insertion	Head of the fibula.
Action	Extends the hip, flexes the knee and internally (medially) rotates the hip.
Antagonist	Quadriceps.
Innervation	long head: Tibial nerve L5-S2 / Short head: Common fibular nerve L5-S2.
Blood Supply	Inferior gluteal artery, perforating arteries, popliteal artery.
Daily Use	Walking, running, cycling, swimming, wiping feet on floor matt.
Gym Use	Squats, deadlifts, lunges, step-ups, leg press, hamstring curls, single-leg balances, jumps.

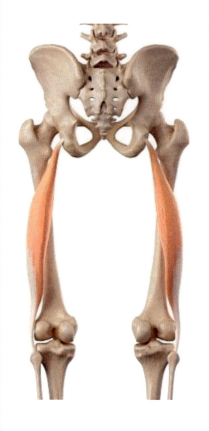

SEMITENDINOSUS

Origin	Ischial tuberosity.
Insertion	Upper medial surface of the tibia – pes anserinus.
Action	Extends the hip, flexes the knee, and posteriorly tilts the pelvis.
Antagonist	Quadriceps.
Innervation	Tibial nerve L5-S2.
Blood Supply	Deep femoral (first perforating branch), medial femoral circumflex, and inferior gluteal arteries.
Daily Use	Walking, running, cycling, swimming, wiping feet on floor matt.
Gym Use	Squats, deadlifts, lunges, step-ups, leg press, hamstring curls, single-leg balances, jumps.

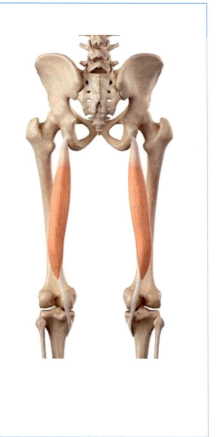

SEMIMEMBRANOSUS	
Origin	Ischial tuberosity.
Insertion	Medial condyloid of the tibia.
Action	Extends the hip, flexes the knee, and posteriorly tilts the pelvis.
Antagonist	Quadriceps.
Innervation	Tibial nerve L5-S2.
Blood Supply	Perforating branches of femoral and popliteal arteries.
Daily Use	Walking, running, cycling, swimming, wiping feet on floor matt.
Gym Use	Squats, deadlifts, lunges, step-ups, leg press, hamstring curls, single-leg balances, jumps.

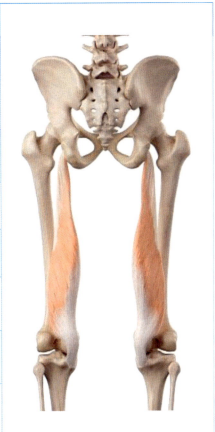

ROLLING THE HAMSTRINGS:

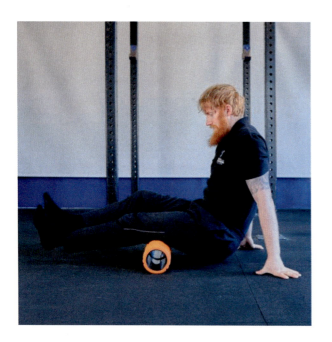

1. Sit on the floor and place a foam roller under the top of your right or left hamstring.
2. Both sides can be done at the same time if the roller is long enough. However, doing one at a time allows for more pressure to be placed through the hamstrings.
3. If rolling your left leg, place your right foot over your left, then raise yourself up with your hands.
4. Slowly roll up and down the muscle for 30-60 seconds. Ensure you do not roll over the back of the knee, as there are structures in your knee crease (lymph nodes) that you don't want to drive a roller into. Focus on the bulk of the muscle.
5. Complete 1-2 times on each side.

BARBELL ROLLING THE HAMSTRINGS:

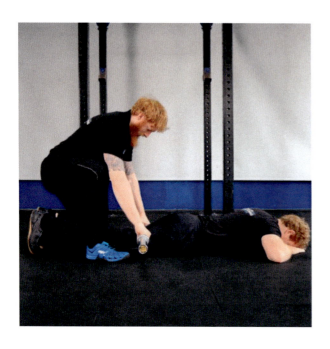

1. Instruct the client to lie on their front.
2. Place a barbell on the hamstrings – use the appropriate load (discomfort not pain).
3. Slowly roll up and down the muscle for 30-60 seconds. Do not roll over the back of the knee, as there are structures in your knee crease that you don't respond well to rolling. Focus on the bulk of the muscle.
4. Complete 1-2 times.

BARBELL ROLLING THE HAMSTRINGS:

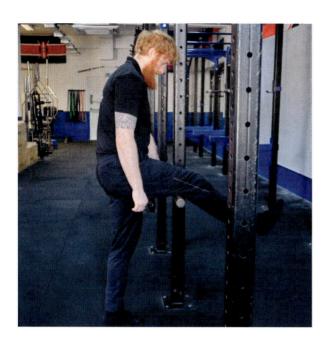

1. Set a barbell up on the rack at around mid-thigh height.
2. Stand in front of the rack so when you place your leg on it, you can easily push it back into the rack/J-cup (as pictured) – this drill can be safely done from either side of the rack.
3. Place your leg over the sleeve to rest your hamstrings on it.
4. Slowly roll up and down the muscle for 30-60 seconds. Do not roll over the back of the knee, as there are structures in your knee crease that you don't respond well to rolling. Focus on the bulk of the muscle.
5. Complete 1-2 times on each side.

HIGH HAMSTRING RELEASE:

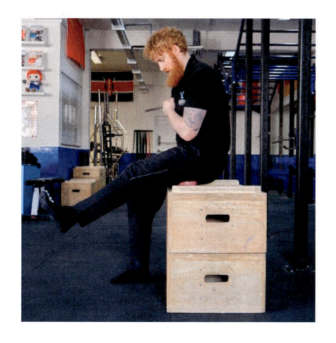

1. Place the massage ball on a solid chair or platform.
2. Sit on the ball so that it is driven into the top of your hamstrings.
3. Knead the soft tissues and find any areas of excessive tension.
4. Apply pressure to an area of tension and slowly straighten and bend the knee.
5. Complete 1-2 sets of 5-10 reps on each leg.

BILATERAL HAMSTRING STRETCH:

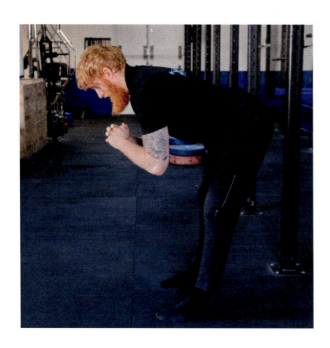

1. Stand with your feet hip-width or slightly wider apart.
2. Keep your knees straight throughout. However, they do not have to be locked out – you can maintain a soft knee position (slight bend).
3. Hinge at your hips by driving your glutes back, ensuring your knees do not bend and your chest remains proud.
4. As your glutes move back, you will feel the stretch on your hamstrings.
5. Hold for 30-60 seconds, or 2 minutes if the musculature is very tense.
6. Complete 1-3 times.

UNILATERAL HAMSTRING STRETCH:

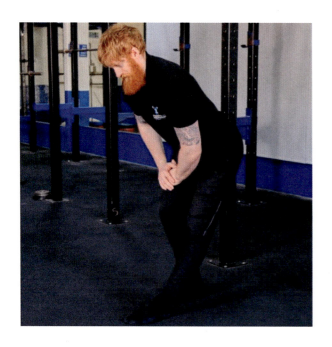

1. Stand in a hip-width stance and place one foot to the front – keep the sole of your foot flat.
2. Bend the rear leg and sit back with your glutes to increase the stretch.
3. Raising your toes off the floor will increase the stretch and place far more emphasis on the calves.
4. Hold for 30-60 seconds, or 2 minutes if the musculature is very tense.
5. Complete 1-3 times on each side.

WIDE STANCE HAMSTRING STRETCH:

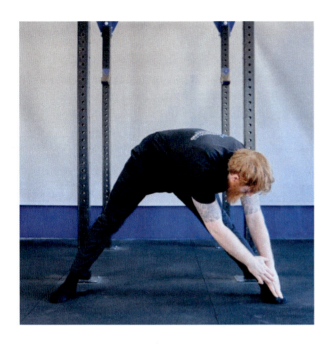

1. Adopt a wide stance.
2. Bend over and reach to one foot to apply the stretch to your hamstrings and adductors – this can be done with a hip hinge and neutral spine, or with a bent spine to increase the stretch through your erectors.
3. Hold for 30-60 seconds, or 2 minutes if the musculature is very tense.
4. Complete 1-3 times.

SEATED HAMSTRING STRETCH:

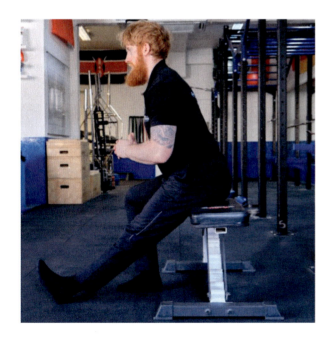

1. Sit at the front of a chair or bench and shift your glutes back slightly, tilting your pelvis forward.
2. Place one or both legs out onto your heel(s).
3. Lean forward with your torso, ensuring you don't round your back – if your pelvis is tilted and your lumbar spine extended (curved inwards) the stretch will be intense.
4. Hold for 30-60 seconds, or 2 minutes if the musculature is very tense.
5. Complete 1-3 times.

FLOOR HAMSTRING STRETCH:

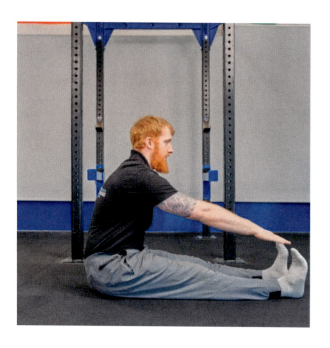

1. Sit on the floor with both legs out to your front.
2. Push your chest out and lean forward (bend at your hips, not your spine) to create a hamstring stretch.
3. You can reach forward with your hands and progress to rounding your spine to stretch your entire posterior chain (muscles that run up the back of your body).
4. Hold for 30-60 seconds, or 2 minutes if the musculature is very tense.
5. Complete 1-3 times.

HURDLER HAMSTRING STRETCH:

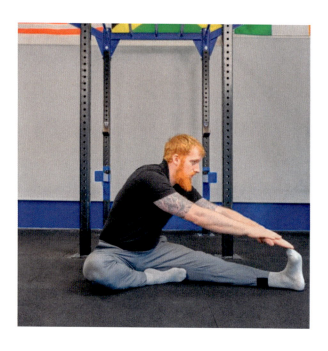

1. Sit on the floor with both legs out to your front.
2. Pull one leg into your groin so that the sole of the foot is pulled into the inner thigh of the straight leg.
3. Push your chest out and lean forward towards the straight leg (bend at your hips, not your spine) to create a hamstring stretch.
4. You can reach forward with your hands and progress to rounding your spine to stretch your entire posterior chain (muscles on the back of your body).
5. Hold for 30-60 seconds, or 2 minutes if the musculature is very tense.
6. Complete 1-3 times on each side.

LYING HAMSTRING STRAP STRETCH:

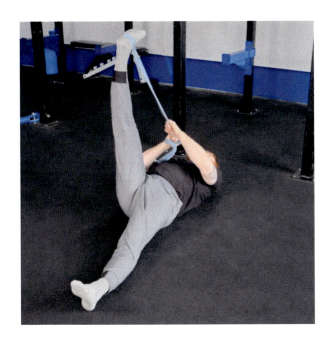

1. Sit on the floor.
2. Place a strap or resistance band around the arch of one foot, holding it with both hands.
3. Lie back, so your head is flat to the floor. Maintain a neutral spine position.
4. Gently pull on the band to raise the leg up to facilitate the stretch.
5. Hold for 30-60 seconds, or 2 minutes if the musculature is very tense.
6. Complete 1-3 times on each side.

DOWNWARD DOG:

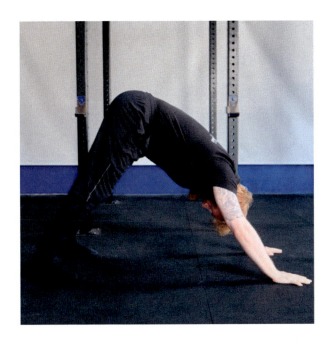

1. Start in a high plank position (plank on your hands), with your shoulders over your wrists and your feet hip-width apart.
2. Raise your hips up to form a pyramid shape. This will result with your head coming between your arms (thoracic extension).
3. There should be a straight line from your hands to your hips, and from your hips to your heels.
4. Straighten your legs and drop your heels towards the floor to increase the stretch on your hamstrings.
5. Hold the position for 30-60 seconds.

LOADED HAMSTRING STRETCH:

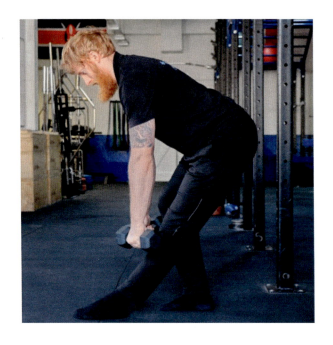

1. Adopt a split stance position with the rear leg bent – your weight should be on the rear leg.
2. Keep the sole of the front foot down to place the emphasis on the hamstrings and raise your toes to increase the stretch on the gastrocnemius.
3. While holding weights (dumbbells/kettlebells), hinge at your hips (sit back with your glutes) to allow the weights to track down your front leg.
4. Ensure you maintain an extended spine.
5. Hold the bottom position for 5-15 seconds and perform 3-5 reps.

PARTNER HAMSTRING PNF:

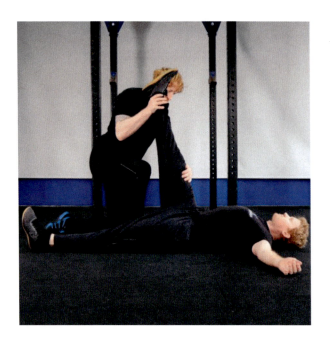

1. Have the client lie on their back.
2. Pick one leg up and place one hand just below their knee (on their thigh) and your other hand just below their heel on their Achilles/lower calf.
3. Raise the leg to the barrier position.
4. Hold the stretch for 10-15 seconds before releasing it slightly and instructing the client to push their leg into your hand.
5. Instruct the client to push with 50-60% intensity for 6-8 seconds.
6. Instruct the client to stop contracting and allow 1-2 seconds for the muscle to relax fully. During this time, instruct the client to take a deep breath in.
7. Instruct the client to exhale slowly, and as they do, push the leg into the next barrier position and hold for 10-15 seconds.
8. Repeat the previous steps 2-3 times and hold the final position for 20-30+ seconds.
9. Complete the stretch on both sides.

SOLO HAMSTRING PNF:

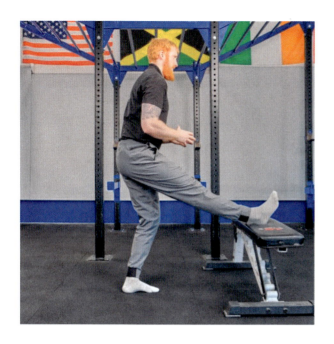

1. Stand and place one heel onto a box/bench (around 20 inches high).
2. Keep your chest proud and lean forward to feel the stretch through your hamstrings.
3. Hold the stretch for 10-15 seconds before releasing it slightly and pushing your heel into the box/bench – 50-60% intensity for 6-8 seconds.
4. Stop contracting, take a deep breath in, and allow 1-2 seconds for the muscle to relax fully.
5. Exhale slowly and lean forward again to apply the stretch and into the next barrier position and hold for 10-15 seconds.
6. Repeat the previous steps 2-3 times and hold the final position for 20-30+ seconds.
7. Complete the stretch on both sides.

BAND HAMSTRING CURL:

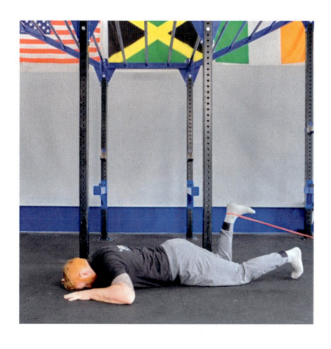

1. Attach a low-tension band to a solid structure.
2. Loop the band around one or both legs (you can loop the band 2-3 times).
3. Turn away from the band and lie on your front.
4. Engage your hamstrings to flex your knees.
5. Complete 2-3 sets of 10-20 reps.

EXERCISE BALL HAMSTRING CURL:

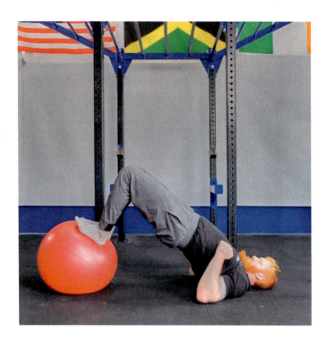

1. Take an exercise ball and lie on your back.
2. Place your calves onto the ball and raise your body up so you are supported by your upper back and your legs on the ball.
3. Pull your heels in towards your glutes.
4. One or both legs can be used.
5. Complete 2-3 sets of 10-20 reps.

BAND GOOD MORNING:

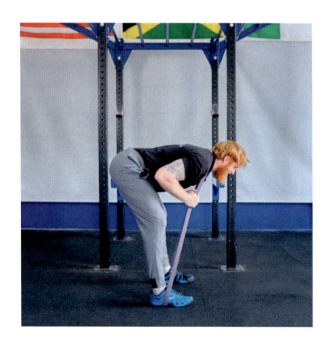

1. Stand inside of a medium to high tension band.
2. Hinge at your hips and place the band over the back of your neck.
3. Explosively extend your hips to stand up straight.
4. Hinge at your hips until your torso is just above parallel to the floor – maintain soft knees and ensure your glutes push rearwards to maximize the stretch and activation of the hamstrings.
5. Perform 2-3 sets of 10-20 reps.

THE TENSOR FASCIAE LATAE (TFL)

The tensor fasciae latae (TFL) is located on the outside of your upper thigh and attaches to the iliotibial band (ITB), along with the gluteus maximus.

The ITB is a sheet of fascia which runs down your outer thigh from your hip to just below your knee and, along with the muscles that connect into it, it plays a role in stabilizing your hip and knee.

When experiencing pain, it's common for people to zone in on the specific area of discomfort immediately. Often, the problem results from other areas of tension or imbalance. It's usually worth considering the areas directly above and below, or either side of the site of pain. Rolling the ITB may alleviate some outer leg pain in the short-term, but it is often overused and has minimal long-term benefits.

Discomfort on the outer side of your leg can be helped by strengthening your leg's supporting muscles, such as your gluteus medius, and releasing the muscles that can take up the slack when the glutes are not pulling their weight, such as the TFL.

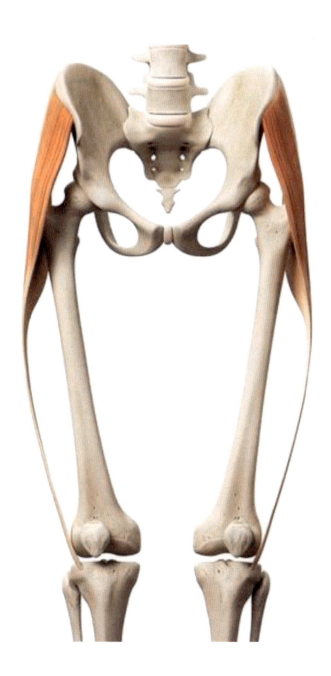

TENSOR FASCIAE LATAE	
Origin	Anterior iliac crest.
Insertion	Lateral upper tibia via iliotibial band (ITB).
Action	Flexes and abducts the hip.
Antagonist	Adductors.
Innervation	Superior gluteal nerve L4-S1.
Blood Supply	Lateral circumflex femoral artery.
Daily Use	Walking, running, swimming.
Gym Use	Squats, deadlifts, lunges, step-ups, single-leg balances, jumps.

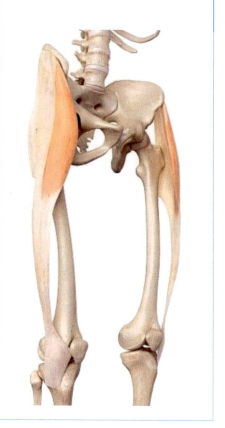

ROLLING THE TFL:

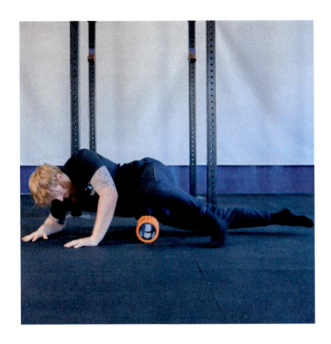

1. Lie on the foam roller with the outer side of your hip, directly where your pants pocket would be.
2. Bring your other leg to the front and place your foot down in line with the knee of the leg being rolled for support.
3. Use your forearm and hand to support yourself.
4. Slowly roll up and down the muscle for 30-60 Seconds.
5. Repeat on both sides.
6. Complete 1-2 sets on each side.

TFL STRETCH:

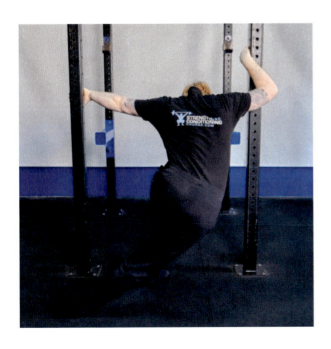

1. Stand in a hip-width stance and hold onto a solid structure.
2. To stretch your right TFL, take your right leg, bring it behind your left leg, and reach as far as you can towards the left.
3. Once you have reached as far as you can with your right leg and the outer side of your right foot is on the floor, push your body weight to the right and down to apply the stretch – having support allows you to increase the ROM without risking injury.
4. Hold for 30-60 seconds, or 2 minutes if the musculature is very tense.
5. Complete 1-3 times on each side.

THE GLUTEALS

The three muscles of the glutes (gluteus maximus, medius, and minimus) can become tense and benefit significantly from release techniques.

The piriformis is a small muscle located under your gluteus maximus. The sciatic nerve travels either underneath or through the piriformis.

The piriformis can become tense through overwork while running, especially if your main gluteal muscles don't pull their weight.

When the piriformis becomes tense, it can be a literal pain in your butt, and the location of your sciatic nerve can result in sciatic pain that shoots down the leg from the lower back.

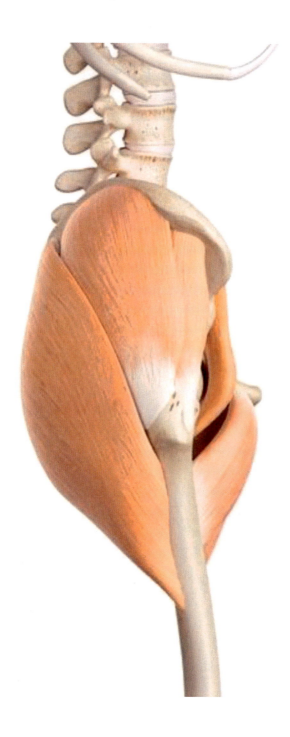

GLUTEUS MAXIMUS

Origin	Coccyx, sacrum and iliac crest.
Insertion	Upper femur and iliotibial band (ITB).
Action	Extends, abducts, and externally (laterally) rotates the hip.
Antagonist	Hip flexors.
Innervation	Inferior gluteal nerve L5-S2.
Blood Supply	Superior and inferior gluteal arteries.
Daily Use	Walking, running, swimming.
Gym Use	Squats, deadlifts, hip thrusts, lunges, step-ups, leg press, single-leg balances, jumps.

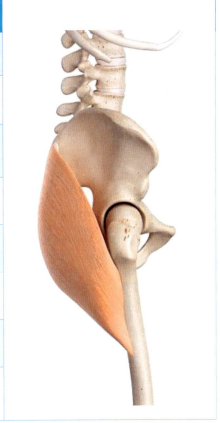

GLUTEUS MEDIUS

Origin	Upper lateral surface of ilium.
Insertion	Lateral surface of greater trochanter.
Action	Abducts the hips. Anterior fibres internally rotate the hips; posterior fibres externally rotate the hip.
Antagonist	Adductors.
Innervation	Superior gluteal nerve L4-S1.
Blood Supply	Superior gluteal artery.
Daily Use	Walking, running, swimming.
Gym Use	Squats, deadlifts, lunges, step-ups, lateral band walks, single-leg balances, jumps.

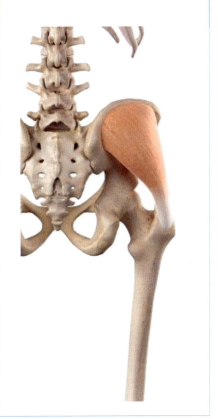

GLUTEUS MINIMUS

Origin	Lateral surface of ilium.
Insertion	Anterior surface of greater trochanter.
Action	Abducts and internally (medially) rotates of the hip.
Antagonist	Adductors.
Innervation	Superior gluteal nerve L4-S1.
Blood Supply	Superior gluteal artery.
Daily Use	Walking, running, swimming.
Gym Use	Squats, deadlifts, lunges, step-ups, lateral band walks, single-leg balances, jumps.

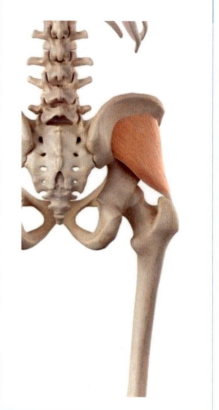

PIRIFORMIS

Origin	Anterior surface of the sacrum.
Insertion	Superior surface of greater trochanter.
Action	Abducts and external rotation of the hip – internally rotates the hip when bent at 90 degrees.
Antagonist	Adductors.
Innervation	Nerve to the piriformis S1-S2.
Blood Supply	Superior gluteal, inferior gluteal, gemellar branches of the internal pudendal arteries.
Daily Use	Walking, running, swimming.
Gym Use	Squats, deadlifts, lunges, step-ups, single-leg balances, jumps.

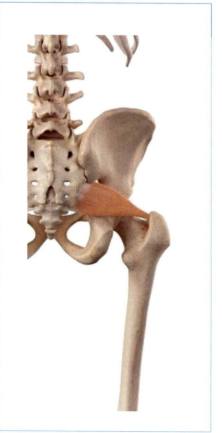

ROLLING THE GLUTEUS MAXIMUS:

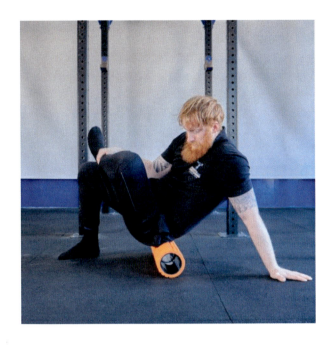

1. Place a foam roller or massage ball on the floor. A foam roller will help distribute the pressure across the gluteal area and be less intense.
2. Place your upper gluteal area on the foam roller (where your back pockets would be).
3. To roll your left-hand side, place your left leg over your right, so your left leg's ankle is just above your right knee. This lengthens the musculature being worked.
4. If this is not possible, simply drop your right knee off to the side.
5. Slowly roll up and down the muscle mass for 30-60 seconds.
6. Complete 1-2 times on each side.

ROLLING THE GLUTEUS MEDIUS/MINIMUS:

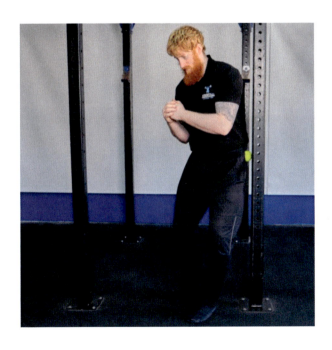

1. Standing: Place the massage ball against a wall at hip height.
2. Lean into the massage ball with the outer side of your glutes.
3. Lying: Place the massage ball onto the floor and lie onto it with the outer side of your glutes.
4. Knead the tissues for 30-60 seconds.
5. Complete 1-2 times on each side.

SEATED (CHAIR) GLUTE STRETCH:

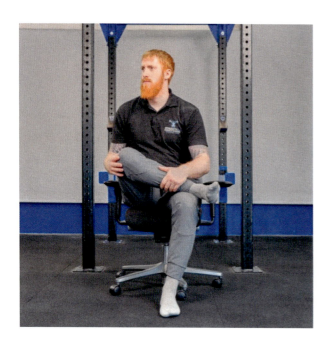

1. Sit upright in your chair/bench.
2. To stretch your right side, place your right leg over your left, so your right leg's ankle is just above your left knee.
3. While keeping your chest proud, lean towards your right knee. Push your chest forward with a neutral spine.
4. Hold for 30-60 seconds, or 2 minutes if the musculature is very tense.
5. Complete 1-3 times on each side.

SEATED (FLOOR) GLUTE STRETCH:

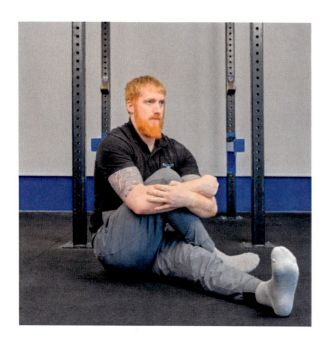

1. Sit on the floor with your legs out to the front.
2. To stretch your left side, raise your left leg and bring it over your right leg – placing your left foot down on the outer side of your right knee.
3. Hug your left leg and pull it towards yourself to stretch the glutes or bring your left arm to the rear (for support) and your right arm across to the outer side of your right leg and push back on the leg.
4. Hold for 30-60 seconds, or 2 minutes if the musculature is very tense.
5. Complete 1-3 times on each side.

FIGURE FOUR GLUTE STRETCH:

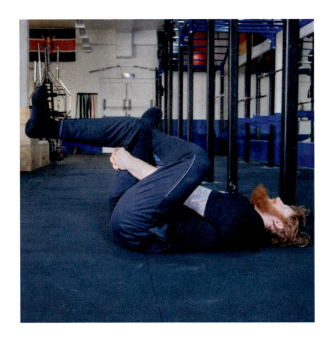

1. Lie on your back.
2. To stretch your left side, raise your right leg up with your knee bent at 90 degrees.
3. Place your left leg over your right, so your left leg's ankle is just below your right knee.
4. Reach through and grab round the back of your right leg with both hands and pull towards your chest.
5. Performing this stretch with the supporting legs foot against a wall (pushing it back) is a great way to increase the intensity of the stretch.
6. Hold for 30-60 seconds, or 2 minutes if the musculature is very tense.
7. Complete 1-3 times on each side.

STANDING GLUTE STRETCH:

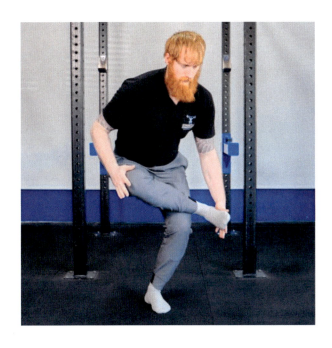

1. Stand upright in a hip-width stance.
2. If stretching your right leg, bring your right foot over your left leg – the outer side of your right ankle should be just above your left knee (bottom of your left thigh).
3. Sit back with your hips to apply the stretch to your glutes.
4. This can be done with or without support (holding onto a post, etc).
5. Hold for 30-60 seconds, or 2 minutes if the musculature is very tense.
6. Complete 1-3 times on each side.

PIGEON GLUTE STRETCH:

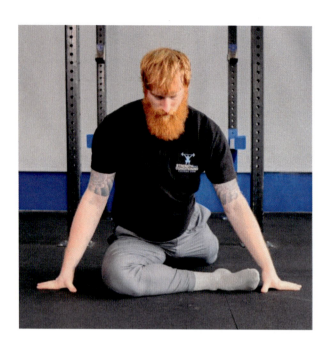

1. Start on all fours.
2. To stretch your right side, place the outer side of your right leg onto the floor. The sole of your right foot will be pointing to the left, while your knee is pointing to the right.
3. Slide your left leg back as you move your right leg into position.
4. Keep your hips forward-facing and your chest proud.
5. Hinge forward while keeping your spine extended to increase the stretch – you can fold (bend) forward to stretch through your back also.
6. If you can, keep your right foot in line with your right knee. However, you might need to pull your foot back towards your hip.
7. Hold for 30-60 seconds, or 2 minutes if the musculature is very tense.
8. Complete 1-3 times on each side.

BOX PIGEON GLUTE STRETCH:

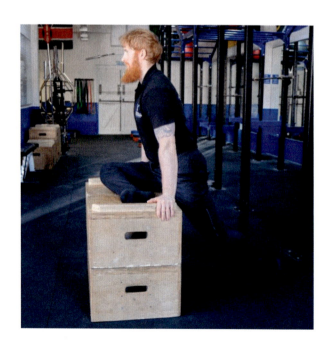

1. Stand behind a box.
2. To stretch your right side, place the outer side of your right leg onto the box. The sole of your right foot will be pointing to the left, while your knee is pointing to the right.
3. Stride back with your left leg as you move your right leg into position.
4. Keep your hips forward-facing and your chest proud.
5. Hinge forward while keeping your spine extended to increase the stretch.
6. If you can, keep your right foot in line with your right knee. However, you might need to pull your foot back towards your hip.
7. Hold for 30-60 seconds, or 2 minutes if the musculature is very tense.
8. Complete 1-3 times on each side.

POSTERIOR BAND DISTRACTION:

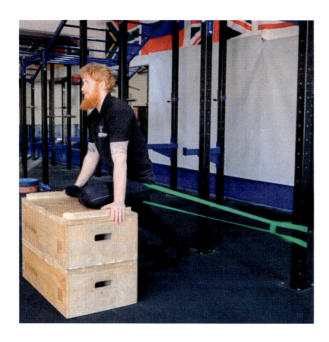

1. Attach a high-tension band around a solid structure.
2. Step into the band and loop it around the top of your leg (pull it right into your groin).
3. Step forward at an oblique angle away from the band attachment point.
4. To stretch your left side, place the outer side of your left leg onto the box.
5. Stride back with your right leg as you move your left leg into position.
6. Keep your hips forward-facing and your chest proud.
7. Hinge forward while keeping your spine extended to increase the stretch.
8. If you can, keep your right foot in line with your right knee. However, you might need to pull your foot back towards your hip.
9. Hold for 30-60 seconds, or 2 minutes if the musculature is very tense.
10. Complete 1-3 times on each side.

GLUTE BRIDGE:

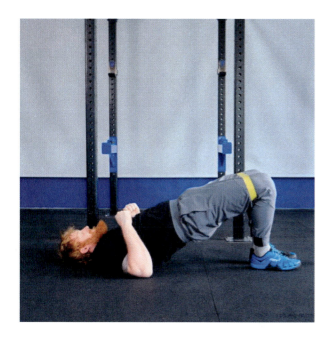

1. Sit on the floor and place a small band around your legs, just above your knees.
2. Lie back, so your head is flat to the floor.
3. Bend your knees and bring your heels towards your glutes. This prevents your hamstrings from taking over the work.
4. Place your feet flat to the floor – coming up onto your heels will increase glute engagement.
5. Spread your knees apart to abduct and externally rotate your hips – increases glute engagement.
6. If performing a single leg glute bridge, extend one of your knees, keeping it in line with the other knee – the supporting leg will have to come in closer towards the midline to balance the movement.
7. Squeeze your glutes and extend your hips.
8. Hold at the top for 1-3 seconds before returning to the starting position.
9. Complete 2-3 sets of 20-30 reps.

HIP THRUST:

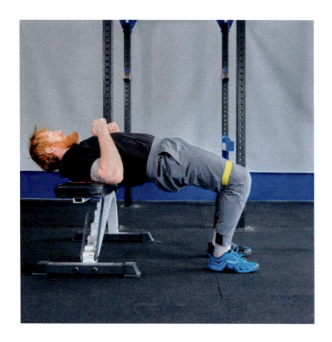

1. Place your mid-back (just below your shoulder blades) onto a bench.
2. Place your hands to the side.
3. Bend your knees and bring your heels towards your glutes. This prevents your hamstrings from taking over the work. However, it is normal for the hamstrings to work alongside the glutes.
4. If performing a single-leg hip thrust, extend one of your knees, keeping it in line with the other knee – the supporting leg will have to come in closer towards the midline to balance the movement.
5. Squeeze your glutes and extend your hips.
6. Hold at the top for 1-3 seconds before returning to the starting position.
7. Complete 2-3 sets of 10-30 reps on each side.

KNEELING HIP THRUST:

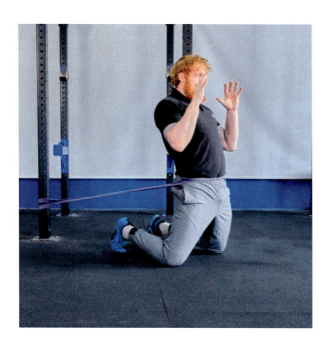

1. Attach a medium to a high-tension resistance band (purple or green) around a solid structure (loop it through itself).
2. Step inside the band so that the band wraps around the crease of your hips.
3. Step forward to apply tension onto the band and kneel on the floor (you can shuffle forward while on your knees to increase the band tension).
4. Hinge at your hips, so the band pulls your glutes rearward.
5. Contract your glutes and bring your hips into full extension.
6. Squeeze your glutes hard at the top.
7. Complete 2-3 sets of 10-20 reps.

PULL THROUGH:

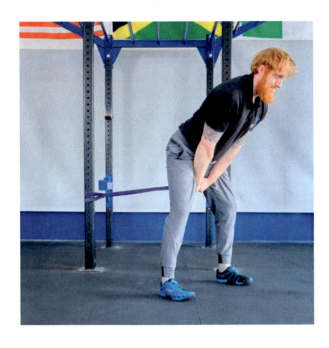

1. Attach a medium to a high-tension resistance band (purple or green) around a solid structure (loop it through itself).
2. Stand with your back towards the band attachment point and hold the end of the band between your legs.
3. Step forward to apply tension to the band.
4. Hinge at your hips, pushing your glutes rearwards. This will result in your arms reaching through your legs and behind you.
5. Holding the band tight in your hands, contract your glutes and bring your hips into full extension.
6. Squeeze your glutes hard at the top.
7. Complete 2-3 sets of 10-20 reps.

DONKEY KICK-BACK:

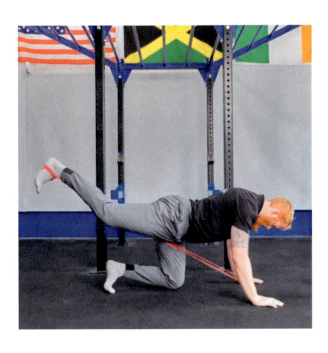

1. Loop a low-tension resistance band around one foot.
2. Loop the other end of the band around your hand (thumb) and place your hand down.
3. Come onto all fours.
4. Kick the foot with the band back, straighten the leg and hyperextend your hip to maximize the glute engagement.
5. Complete 2-3 sets of 10-20 reps on each side.

LATERAL BAND WALK:

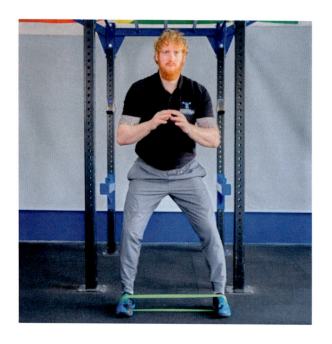

1. Place a small loop band around your feet or lower legs or hold a long band in each hand and stand on it – having it around your feet can help to increase glute engagement.
2. Stand up tall with good posture, bend your knees slightly.
3. Step 1-2 foot-widths in the direction you are going. Stay in control, and don't allow your leg to be dragged by the band.
4. Complete 2-3 sets of 10-20 strides in each direction.

FIRE HYDRANT:

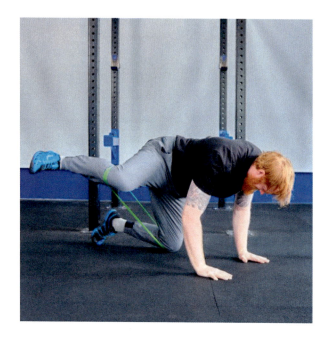

1. Kneel onto all fours (quadruped position).
2. A small loop band can be used to increase the intensity of the exercise. Loop the band around your legs, just above your knees, and clamp the band down under the non-working leg's knee.
3. Begin the exercise by kicking one leg out to the side while maintaining the bent knee position (like a dog lifting its leg).
4. Try to keep your hips level – don't tilt away from the working leg to increase the range of motion (ROM).
5. Squeeze your glutes hard at the top.
6. Bring your leg back down to the starting position (it doesn't have to touch the floor), before going into successive reps.
7. Complete 2-3 sets of 10-20 reps on each side.

THE LOWER BACK

The muscles of the lower back can easily become tense and cause lower (low) back pain.

The "low back" refers to the area between the bottom of your ribs and the bottom of your glutes (lumbo-pelvic region – lumbar spine and pelvis).

A common cause of discomfort in the lower back can be excessive tension in the quadratus lumborum (QL) and/or lower erector spinae. These muscles are located on either side of the spine and attach to your pelvis, so any imbalances here can cause postural issues and have knock-on effects throughout your whole body.

It is generally far more effective to roll each side of the spine independently with a massage ball, either lying on it, or placing it on a wall or a door frame – a long foam roller can result in the lower spine being forced into extension, which can limit the benefits of the release.

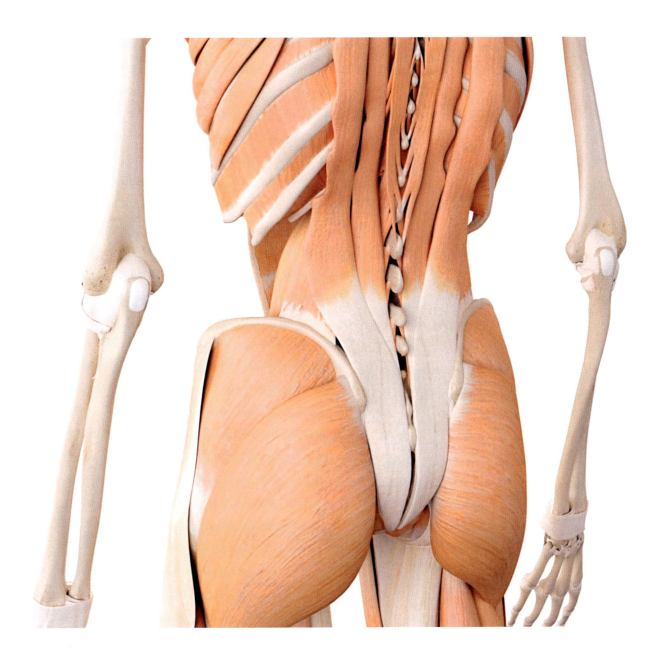

THE ERECOTR SPINAE AND QUADRATUS LUMBORUM

The erector spinae, aka paraspinals, are made up of the iliocostalis, longissimus, and spinalis and run up either side of the spine. Their primary role is extension of the spine.

The quadratus lumborum (QL), just like the erector spinae, are located at either side of the spine. However, rather than running all the way up the spine, they attach between the ilium on the pelvis and the bottom ribs.

The QL's work to extend the spine and also work unilaterally to laterally flex and extend the spine.

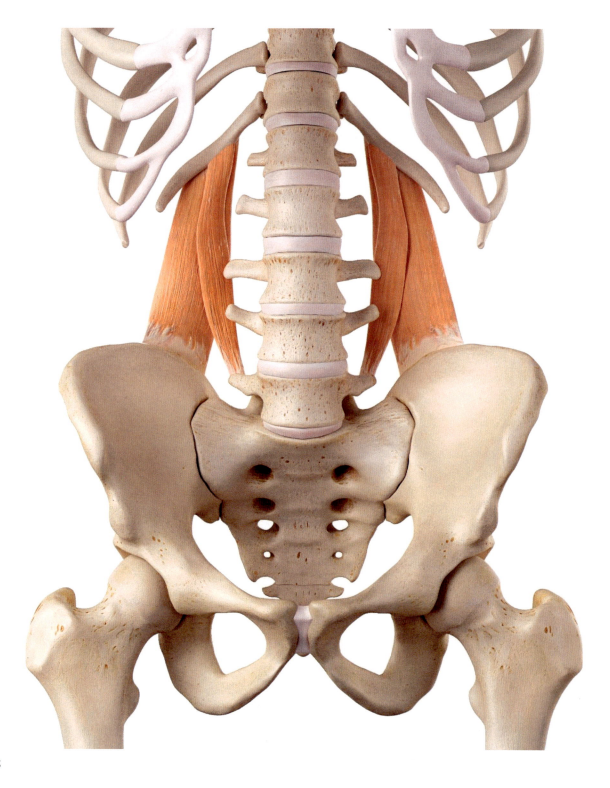

QUADRATUS LUMBORUM

Origin	Posterior iliac crest.
Insertion	12th rib, and transverse processes of L1-L4.
Action	Bilateral: Extends the spine / Unilateral: Laterally flexes and extends the spine and tilts the pelvis.
Antagonist	Abdominals and hip flexors.
Innervation	Subcostal nerve T12, and anterior rami of spinal nerves L1-L4
Blood Supply	Lumbar, median sacral, iliolumbar and subcostal arteries.
Daily Use	Picking up a suitcase. Raising up from a side-lying position.
Gym Use	Deadlifts, dumbbell side bends, side planks.

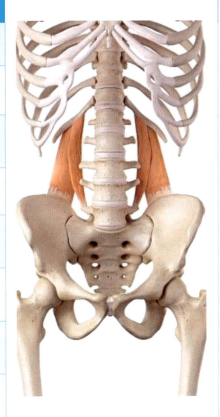

SPINALIS

Origin	Spinous processes: Capitis: C7-T1 / Cervicis: C7-T1 / Thoracis: T11-L2 (Thoracis pictured).
Insertion	Capitis: Occipital bone / Cervicis: Spinous process of C2-C4 / Thoracis: T2-T8
Action	Bilateral: Extends the spine / Unilateral: Laterally flexes and extends the spine.
Antagonist	Abdominals.
Innervation	Lateral branch of posterior rami of spinal nerves.
Blood Supply	Dorsal branch of posterior intercostal, deep cervical, and vertebral arteries.
Daily Use	Maintaining an upright posture and erecting the spine from a bent-over position.
Gym Use	Deadlifts, back extensions.

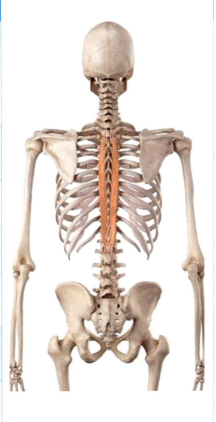

LONGISSIMUS

Origin	Transverse processes of the lumbar and thoracic vertebrae.
Insertion	Ribs and transverse processes of the thoracic and cervical vertebrae, and mastoid process.
Action	Bilateral: Extends the spine / Unilateral: Laterally flexes and extends the spine.
Antagonist	Abdominals.
Innervation	Lateral branches of posterior rami of spinal nerves.
Blood Supply	Sacral, intercostal and subcostal arteries.
Daily Use	Maintaining an upright posture and erecting the spine from a bent-over position.
Gym Use	Deadlifts, back extensions.

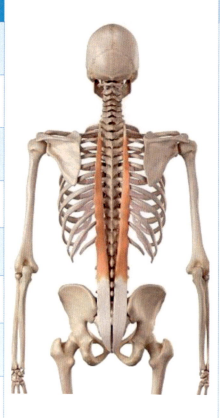

ILIOCOSTALIS

Origin	Sacrum, ilium, and posterior surface of ribs 1-12.
Insertion	Posterior surface of ribs 1-12, and transverse processes of the cervical vertebrae.
Action	Bilateral: Extends the spine / Unilateral: Laterally flexes and extends the spine.
Antagonist	Abdominals.
Innervation	Lateral branches of posterior rami of spinal nerves.
Blood Supply	Sacral, intercostal and subcostal arteries.
Daily Use	Maintaining an upright posture and erecting the spine from a bent-over position.
Gym Use	Deadlifts, back extensions.

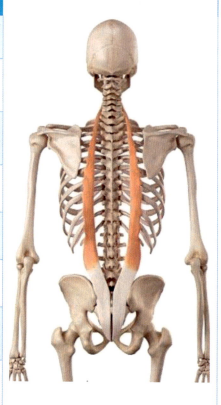

MULTIFIDUS

Origin	Sacrum and transverse processes of lumbar, thoracic, and cervical vertebrae.
Insertion	Spinous processes of 2nd to 4th vertebrae above each origin.
Action	Extends and rotates the spine.
Antagonist	Abdominals.
Innervation	Medial branches of posterior rami of spinal nerves.
Blood Supply	Vertebral, deep cervical, posterior intercostal, subcostal, lumbar and lateral sacral arteries.
Daily Use	Returning from a bending movement. Turning to put on your seatbelt.
Gym Use	Deadlifts, back extensions.

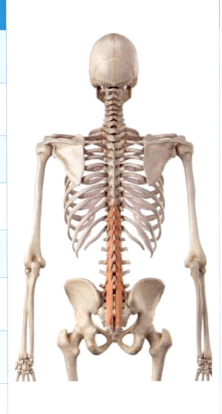

ROTATORES

Origin	Transverse processes of lumbar through cervical vertebrae.
Insertion	Spinous processes of lumbar through to the second cervical vertebra (span 1-2 vertebrae).
Action	Extends and rotates the spine.
Antagonist	Abdominals.
Innervation	Medial branches of posterior rami of spinal nerves.
Blood Supply	Dorsal branches of posterior intercostal and lumbar arteries.
Daily Use	Returning from a bending movement. Turning to put on your seatbelt.
Gym Use	Deadlifts, back extensions.

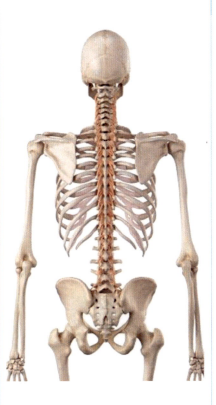

ROLLING THE ERECTORS AND QL'S:

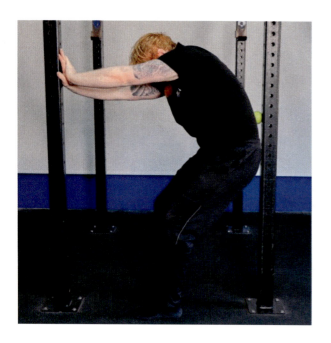

1. Place a massage ball or peanut-shaped ball on the floor if lying on it or against a wall or door frame at hip height.
2. Place the right side of your lower back onto the ball, just above your pelvis.
3. Keep your pelvis neutral or tilted slightly back to drive the soft tissue into the ball.
4. If lying, you can raise the knee of the side you are working, allowing you to drive the ball deeper into the soft tissue.
5. If working in a door frame or similar space, you can push against the structure to the front of you to increase the pressure. Remember, although a lot of pressure on tense lower back muscles, are aim is to stimulate not annihilate.
6. Slowly roll up and down the muscle mass for 30-60 seconds.
7. Complete 1-2 times on each side.

KNEES TO CHEST STRETCH:

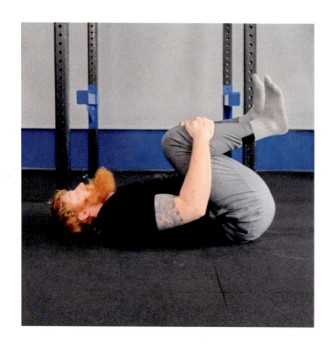

1. Lie on your back.
2. Bring one or both knees up and hug them in your arms to increase the stretch.
3. Hold for 30-60 seconds, or 2 minutes if the musculature is very tense.
4. Complete 1-3 times on each side.

HIP ROLL STRETCH:

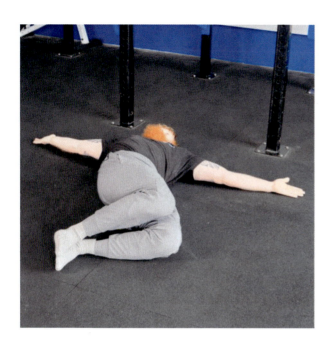

1. Lie on your back with your head flat to the floor, and your arms spread to your sides.
2. Bend your knees so your soles are flat on the floor.
3. Slowly roll your knees side to side while keeping both arms flat to the floor.
4. Complete 2-3 sets of 10-20 rolls.

IRON CROSS STRETCH:

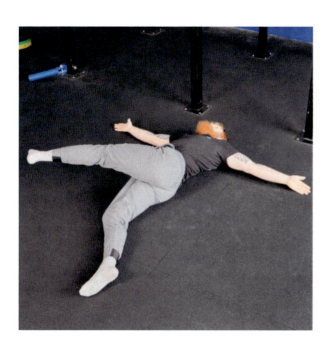

1. Lie on your back with your head flat to the floor, and your arms spread to your sides.
2. While keeping the other leg flat to the floor, slowly raise one leg and bring it towards your opposite hand.
3. Hold this position for 2-3 seconds before returning to the starting position and continuing with the opposite leg.
4. Complete 2-3 sets of 10 reps.

LYING QL STRETCH:

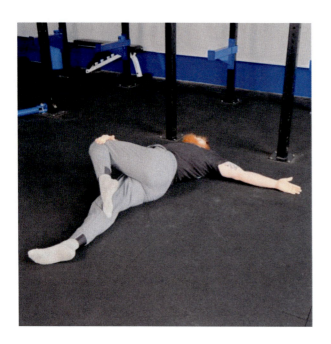

1. Lie on your back with your head flat to the floor, and your arms spread to your sides.
2. To stretch your left side, raise your left leg with a bent knee and bring your right arm across to hold the outer side of your left leg.
3. Your left foot can be placed behind your right knee or your whole leg can be brought over your right leg.
4. Pull your left leg across your body and towards the floor.
5. Ensure your left arm stays flat to the floor as you pull your left leg across to the floor.
6. Hold for 30-60 seconds, or 2 minutes if the musculature is very tense.
7. Complete 1-3 times on each side.

STANDING QL/LOWER ERECTOR STRETCH:

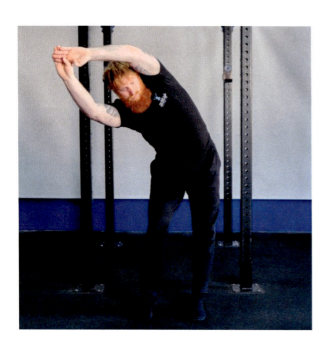

1. Stand upright in a hip-width stance.
2. Take your arms overhead (hands together) and lean to one side.
3. Lean forward slightly to increase the stretch on the QL and lower erectors.
4. Hold for 30-60 seconds, or 2 minutes if the musculature is very tense.
5. Complete 1-3 times on each side.

HOLDING QL/LOWER ERECTOR STRETCH:

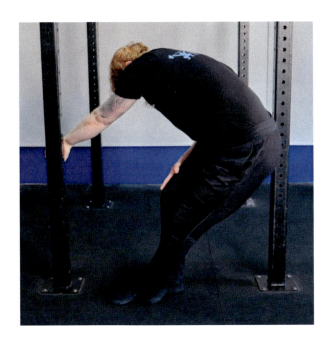

1. Bend over diagonally to your front and allow your spine to flex.
2. Hold onto a solid structure (low) with one arm – this is often best done with the arm on the side you are stretching.
3. Push away with the hip on the side of the QL/erector you are looking to stretch.
4. Hold for 30-60 seconds, or 2 minutes if the musculature is very tense.
5. Complete 1-3 times on each side.

FORWARD BEND STRETCH:

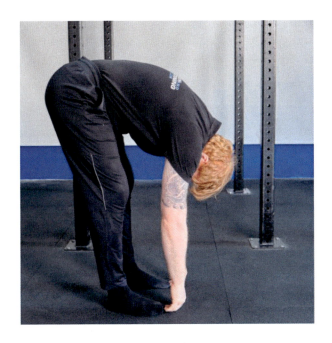

1. Stand up straight in a hip-width stance (the stance width can be modified to suit).
2. Bend forward and drop your arms and torso towards the floor. This is often done slowly "vertebrae by vertebrae".
3. You can fluidly move your hands from your right heel to your left heel in a semicircle pattern to increase the stretch from one side of the lower back to the next.
4. Hold for 30-60 seconds, or 2 minutes if the musculature is very tense.
5. Complete 1-3 times.

DORSAL RAISES:

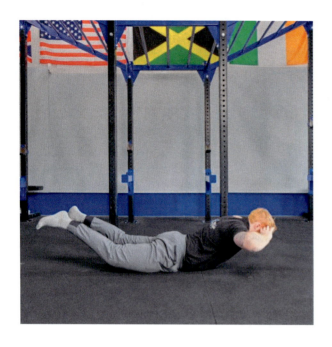

1. Lie on your front.
2. Place your hands at your temples.
3. Engage your back and glute muscles to raise your chest off the floor.
4. You can also raise your legs off the floor at the same time.
5. Complete 2-3 sets of 10-20 reps.

GHD BACK EXTENSIONS:

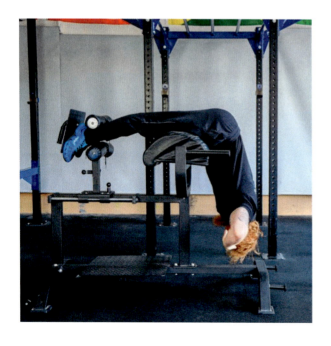

1. Set yourself up on the GHD so that feet are securely through the supports and placed onto the back plate.
2. Your thighs should be supported on the pads and the crease of your hips should be in front of the pads to allow your torso to drop forward.
3. Bend at your hips to drop your torso.
4. Engage the muscles of your posterior chain to raise your torso up.
5. You can stay neutral at the top or hyperextend to maximize the engagement of your back muscles.
6. Complete 2-3 sets of 10-20 reps.

THE MID-UPPER BACK

The middle-upper back's major muscles include the trapezius, rhomboids, latissimus dorsi, and teres major, which is commonly referred to as the "little lat."

The trapezius will be looked at when we get to the neck section.

Other muscles include some of the rotator cuff muscles (external rotators). However, these will be covered in the shoulder section.

We will first look at how we can mobilize the thoracic spine and the specific muscles surrounding it.

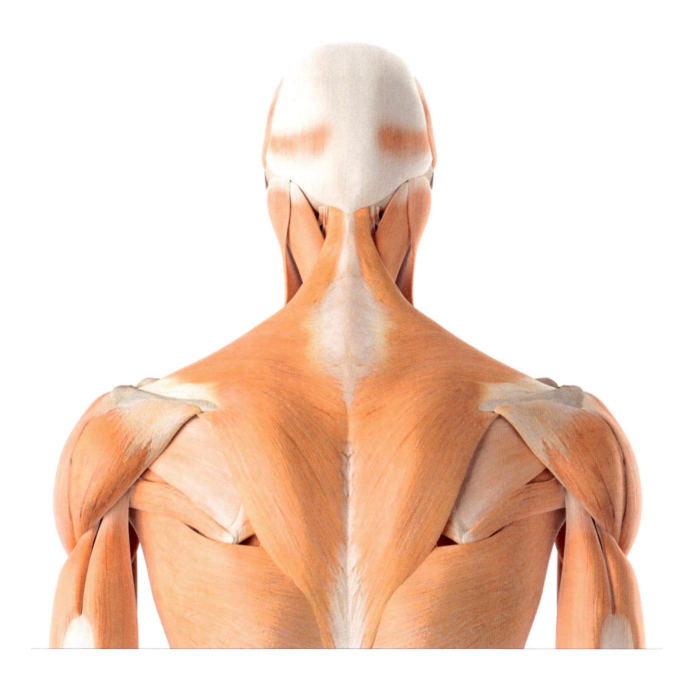

THE THORACIC SPINE

The thoracic spine is made up of 12 vertebrae and is an area that is commonly restricted through both extension and rotation.

Thoracic mobility is extremely important for both upper back and shoulder health and will allow an athlete to perform an overhead press and overhead squat without placing excessive stress on the shoulders and lower spine.

The lumbar spine has some ability to rotate. However, when performing large rotational actions, your thoracic spine and hips should do most of the work. A great visualization is to imagine that you are rotating with your chest.

A greater ROM is achieved when you rotate with both your thoracic spine and hips. However, in this section, we want to isolate thoracic rotation to help mobilize the area.

As mentioned in the posture chapter, during daily activities, movement should primarily come from your limbs, with your torso helping to stabilize these actions. If you initiate movements time and time again through bending and rotating your spine, the risk of future back issues is greatly increased.

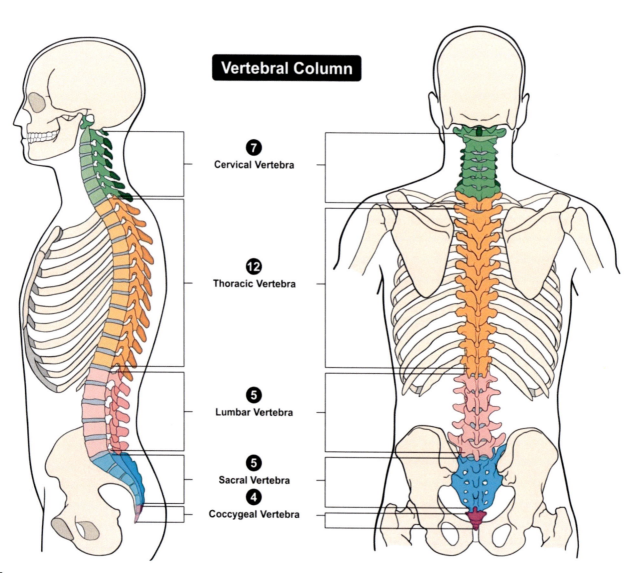

Vertebral Column

7 Cervical Vertebra

12 Thoracic Vertebra

5 Lumbar Vertebra

5 Sacral Vertebra

4 Coccygeal Vertebra

ROLLING THE THORACIC SPINE:

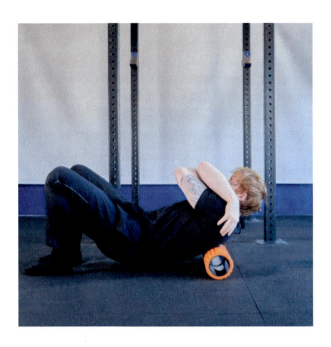

1. Lie with your mid-back on the foam roller.
2. Extend your arms out in front of you and cross them over each other. You want your shoulders protracted (pushed forward) to lengthen the muscles of the back.
3. Slowly roll your mid-upper back area (up and down) for 30-60 seconds.
4. For a great extension drill, keep the foam roller static and take your arms extended overhead. From there, allow gravity to do the work and mobilize each vertebra (holding for 30-60 seconds).
5. Complete 1-2 times on each side.

BARBELL THORACIC EXTENSIONS:

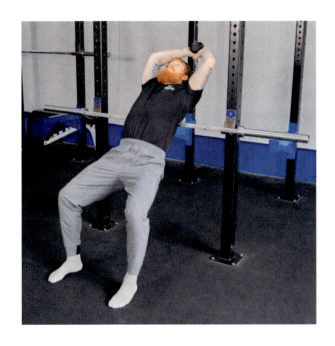

1. Set a barbell up on a rack at hip height.
2. Crouch down and place your mid-back on the barbell, just below your shoulder blades.
3. Raise your hands overhead. You can do this without weight or with a dumbbell in your hands.
4. Exercise caution with the drill. If the stretch becomes too much and you can't raise the weight back overhead, simply drop it.
5. Hold the position for 30-60 seconds and allow gravity to do its work.

CAT-CAMEL:

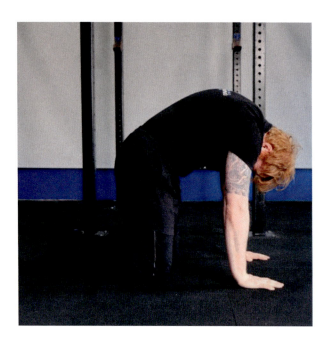

1. Start on all fours with your shoulders over your wrists and your hips over your knees.
2. Look up and extend your entire spine (inward curve – dip your spine).
3. Flex your spine (round your spine), pushing your head down and tucking your buttocks in.
4. Smoothly transition between the extended (cat) and flexed (camel) position.
5. Completed 2-3 sets of 5-10 reps.

STANDING THORACIC ROTATION:

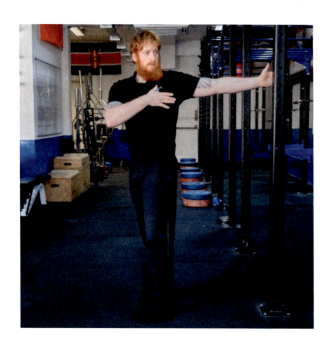

1. Stand up and rotate to one side with your thoracic spine (rotate with your chest).
2. If you are stand in front of the corner of a wall or a post, you can use this to increase the stretch.
3. Hold the stretch for 30-60 seconds, or 2 minutes if the musculature is very tense.
4. Complete 1-3 times on each side.

SEATED THORACIC ROTATION:

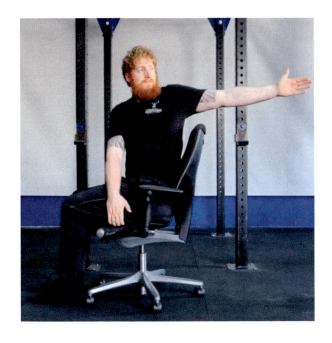

1. Sit in a chair.
2. Reach across your body with your right hand and grab under the left side of your seat.
3. Rotate to the left with your thoracic spine and extend your left arm out behind you.
4. Hold the stretch for 30-60 seconds, or 2 minutes if the musculature is very tense.
5. Complete 1-3 times on each side.

QUADRUPED THORACIC ROTATION:

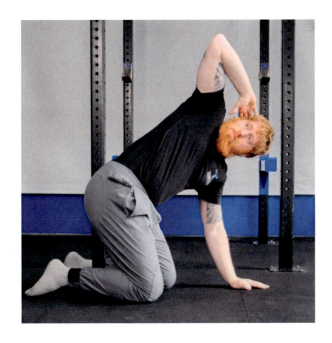

1. Get down onto all fours.
2. Place your right hand behind your head.
3. Shifting back with your hips facilitates a small degree of lumbar flexion, which will take away the arch. This ensures you don't compensate for the movement by rotating your lumbar spine.
4. Place your right elbow under your torso before rotating round and pointing it toward the ceiling or as far as your mobility will allow.
5. Follow your elbow with your eyes.
6. Complete 2-3 sets of 5-10 rotations on each side.

SIDE-LYING THORACIC ROTATION:

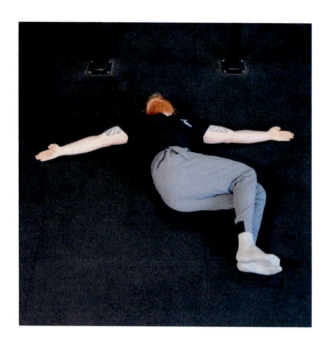

1. Lie on your side.
2. Raise both legs up to 90 degrees.
3. Place your hands out to the front in a prayer position.
4. Slowly rotate with your thoracic spine to bring the top arm over so that the back of your hand touches the floor or as far as mobility allows.
5. Keep your leg firmly on the foam roller throughout the whole movement.
6. Complete 2-3 sets of 5-10 rotations on each side.

BAND ROTATION:

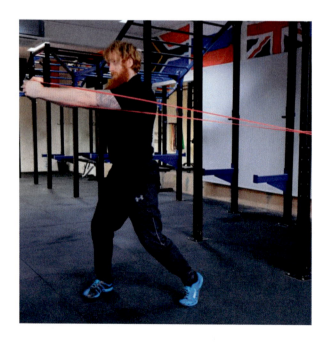

1. Use low-tension resistance band. The tension can be varied by standing closer to or further away from the band attachment point if required.
2. Attach the band to something solid at chest height, looping the band through itself – the band can be attached low, up high, or somewhere in between.
3. Grasp the band with both hands and stand side-on to the attachment point, holding your hands at your chest.
4. Sidestep away from the attachment point to add tension to the band.
5. Rotate away from the attachment point and vary the angles at which your rotate.
6. Complete 2-3 sets of 10 reps on each side.

WOOD-CHOP:

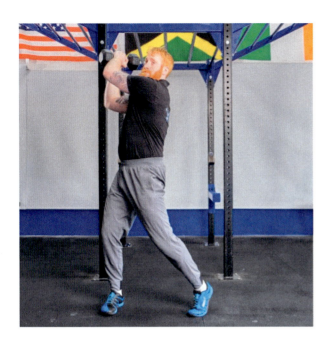

1. Grab a free weight (dumbbell, weight plate, etc) with both hands.
2. Stand in a hip-width to shoulder-width stance.
3. You can swing the weight in any direction, either isolating the rotation to your spine or pivoting on your feet and rotating your hips.
4. You can rotate the weight from side to side or from your knees to over your shoulder and vice versa.
5. Complete 2-3 sets of 10-20 rotations.

THE LATISSIMUS DORSI

The latissimus dorsi (lats) is the broadest muscle on the back - the word latissimus dorsi comes from Latin and means "broadest of the back."

The lats flex and adduct the shoulders.

When the lats become tense, they restrict your ability to take your arms overhead and will negatively impact your overhead press/push press, overhead squat and even your front rack position for the front rack/clean.

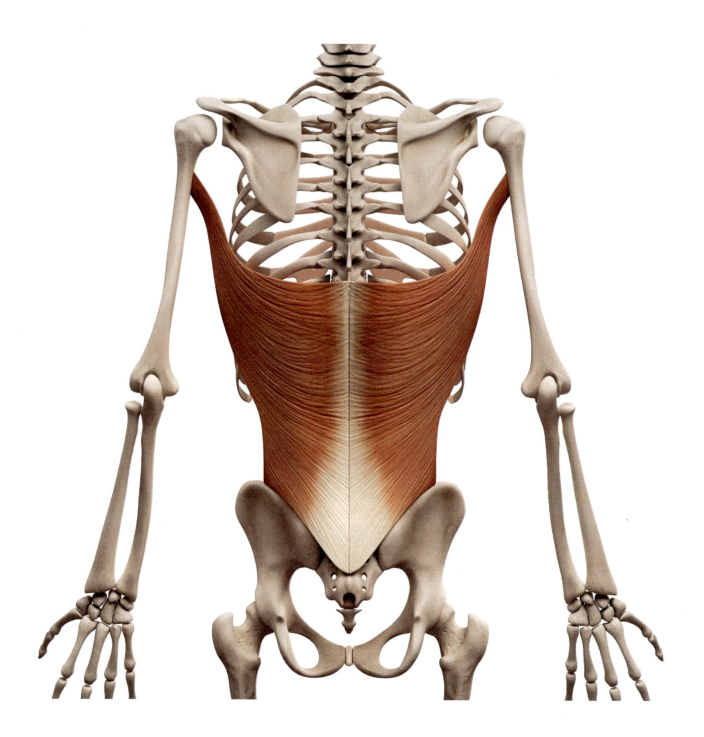

LATISSIMUS DORSI

Origin	Lower 7 thoracic vertebrae, inferior angle of the scapula, thoracolumbar fascia and iliac crest.
Insertion	Anterior upper humerus.
Action	Extends, adducts and internally rotates the shoulder.
Antagonist	Deltoid and trapezius.
Innervation	Thoracodorsal nerve C6-C8.
Blood Supply	Thoracodorsal artery.
Daily Use	Climbing a wall, swimming.
Gym Use	Pull-up, lat pull down, deadlift.

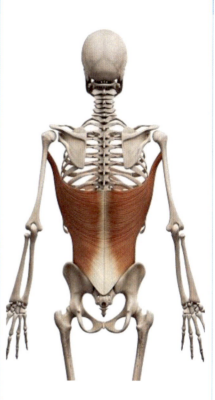

ROLLING THE LATS:

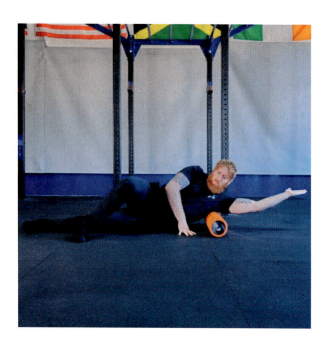

1. Sit down on the floor with the foam roller to your left side.
2. Raise your left arm up and lie down on your side, with the foam roller placed onto the latissimus dorsi. You will feel the large muscle mass just below and to the rear of your armpit.
3. Slowly roll up and down the muscle mass for 30-60 seconds.
4. Complete 1-2 times on each side.

BARBELL ROLLING THE LATS:

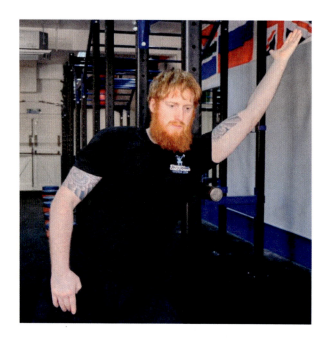

1. Set a barbell up on the rack at lower chest height
2. Stand in front the rack so when you push your lat into the barbell, it pushes it back into the rack/J-cup (as pictured).
3. Raise one arm up with your palm supinated (palm up) and place it onto the sleeve of the barbell.
4. Slowly roll up and down the muscle for 30-60 seconds.
5. Complete 1-2 times on each side.

STANDING LAT STRETCH:

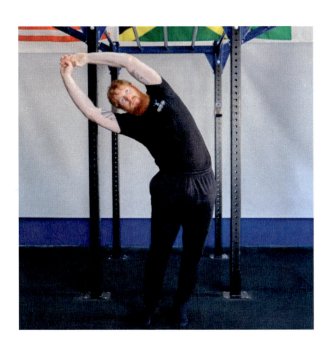

1. Raise your left arm overhead and lean over to your right side. You can bring your right hand up to pull on your left hand slightly.
2. Lean to your right side and forwards while pushing your left hip back. Explore this position to get the best stretch.
3. If you have something solid such as a doorway to hold onto with your left hand as you drive your hips back and rotate your back away from the structure, it will increase the stretch.
4. Hold for 30-60 seconds for a regular stretch, or 2 minutes if the musculature is very tense.
5. Complete 1-3 times on each side.

KNEELING LAT STRETCH (CHILDS POSE):

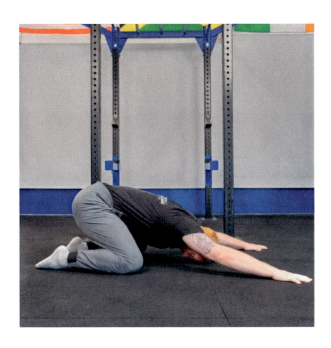

1. Get onto all fours with your hands placed to your front with your palms flat to the floor.
2. Sit back, so your glutes come back towards your heels.
3. Move your hands into the position that facilitates the best stretch. Keep your elbows locked out and spread your fingers.
4. Slowly allow your head to drop between your arms (extend your thoracic spine).
5. Hold for 30-60 seconds for a regular stretch, or 2 minutes if the musculature is very tense.
6. Complete 1-3 times on each side.

DEAD HANG STRETCH:

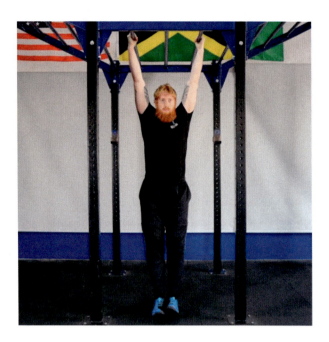

1. Hold onto a bar overhead – this can be done in a pronated (overhand – palms facing away from you), supinated (underhand – palms facing you) or neutral (palms facing each other) grip position.
2. Hang from the bar.
3. You can keep your shoulder blades retracted or allow your shoulder joint to distract to greatly increase the stretch.
4. Pushing your feet to the front slightly (with straight legs), will engage your hip flexors and abdominals and stabilise you position.
5. If height allows, this position can also be done with slight support from you heels on the floor.
6. Hold the position for 5-30 seconds.
7. Complete 1-3 sets.

RESISTANCE BAND LAT STRETCH:

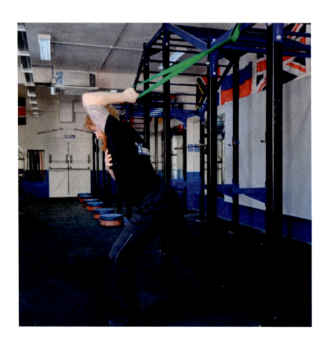

1. Attach the band to something solid, a vertical or horizontal bar is ideal.
2. Grab the band with your left hand, then turn your back to the band, so your arm is bent over your shoulder with your elbow pointing forward and up.
3. Step forward with your left leg and lean forward slightly to put tension onto the band.
4. The band tension will pull back on your arm, creating a great stretch.
5. Be sure not to lean too far forward, as you could lose balance and injure your arm.
6. Hold for 30-60 seconds for a regular stretch, or 2 minutes if the musculature is very tense.
7. Complete 1-3 times on each side.

LOADED LAT STRETCH:

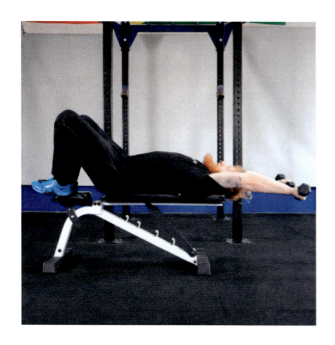

1. Grab a set of light dumbbells and lie on a bench.
2. Bending your knees and raising your feet up onto the bench will flatten your lower spine and prevent it from extending to compensate.
3. With straight arms, bring your arms overhead.
4. Hold the bottom position for 5-15 seconds and perform 3-5 reps.
5. If it gets too heavy, you can simply drop the weights (the weight should be more than manageable).

SOLO (BAND) LAT PNF:

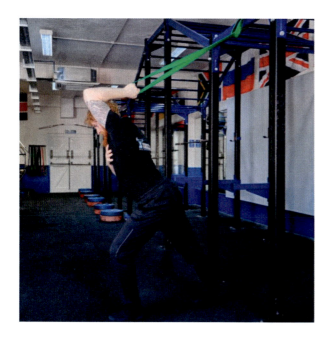

1. Attach the band to something solid, a vertical or horizontal bar is ideal.
2. Grab the band with your left hand, then turn your back to the band, so your arm is bent over your shoulder with your elbow pointing forward and up.
3. Step forward with your left leg and lean forward slightly to put tension onto the band.
4. Hold the stretch for 10-15 seconds before releasing it slightly and pulling on the band to engage the lats – 50-60% intensity for 6-8 seconds.
5. Stop contracting, take a deep breath in, and allow 1-2 seconds for the muscle to relax fully.
6. Exhale slowly and lean forward again to apply the stretch to reach the next barrier position and hold for 10-15 seconds.
7. Repeat the previous steps 2-3 times and hold the final position for 20-30+ seconds.
8. Complete the stretch on both sides.

SOLO STANDING LAT PNF:

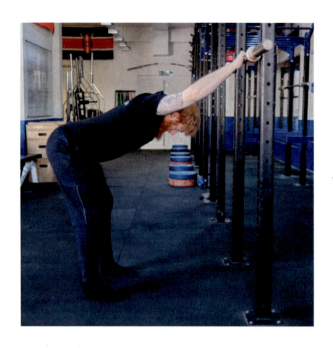

1. Stand behind a barbell on a rack or a windowsill, etc.
2. Place your hands (palms down) onto the barbell.
3. Push your head and torso down to apply the lat stretch (this is a great thoracic extension drill).
4. Hold the stretch for 10-15 seconds before releasing it slightly and push your hands into the barbell to engage the lats – 50-60% intensity for 6-8 seconds.
5. Stop contracting, take a deep breath in, and allow 1-2 seconds for the muscle to relax fully.
6. Exhale slowly, drop your head and torso again to apply the stretch reach the next barrier position, and hold for 10-15 seconds.
7. Repeat the previous steps 2-3 times and hold the final position for 20-30+ seconds.

SOLO KNEELING LAT PNF:

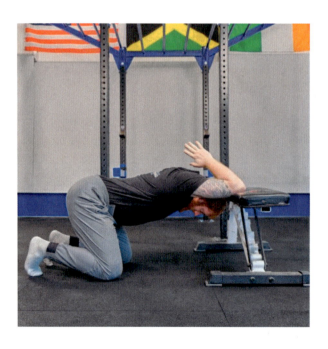

1. Kneel behind a bench/box/sofa.
2. Bend your elbows and bring your hands behind your head – you can put your hands into a prayer position.
3. Lean forward and place the bottom of your upper arms on the bench.
4. Push your head and torso down to apply the lat stretch (this is a great thoracic extension drill).
5. Hold the stretch for 10-15 seconds before releasing it slightly and push your arms into the bench to engage the lats – 50-60% intensity for 6-8 seconds.
6. Stop contracting, take a deep breath in, and allow 1-2 seconds for the muscle to relax fully.
7. Exhale slowly, drop your head and torso again to apply the stretch reach the next barrier position, and hold for 10-15 seconds.
8. Repeat the previous steps 2-3 times and hold the final position for 20-30+ seconds.

LAT PULL DOWN:

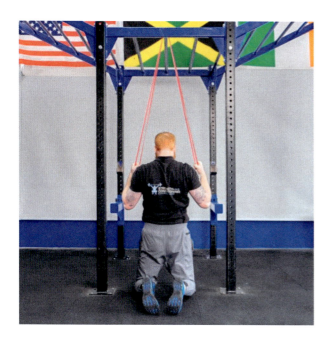

1. Use a low to medium-tension resistance band and attach it up high on a solid structure.
2. Grab each end of the band and kneel or sit down on the floor.
3. Engage your lats and pull down on the band.
4. Bring the band back up to the starting position before continuing with successive reps.
5. Complete 2-3 sets of 10-20 reps.

STRAIGHT-ARM LAT PULL DOWN:

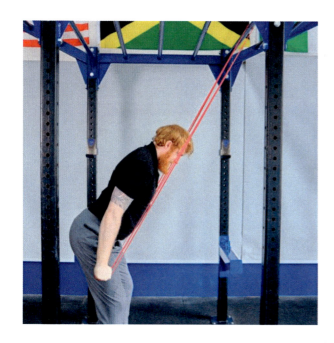

1. Use a low-tension resistance band and attach it up high on a solid structure.
2. Grab each end of the band and walk away from the attachment point to apply tension to the band. At this point, your arms should be straight out to your front or slightly overhead.
3. In this position, you can either stand upright, hinge your hips, or even take a kneeling position.
4. While maintaining straight arms, pull your arms down using your lats until your arms are at your sides.
5. Bring the band back up to the starting position before continuing with successive reps.
6. Complete 2-3 sets of 10-20 reps.

THE RHOMBOIDS

The rhomboids attach between the spine and the scapula (shoulder blades).

The rhomboids are made up between the rhomboids major and the rhomboids minor.

It is not uncommon for individuals to feel tension and discomfort between their shoulder blades. Therefore, the right strength and flexibility techniques to specifically target the rhomboids are key.

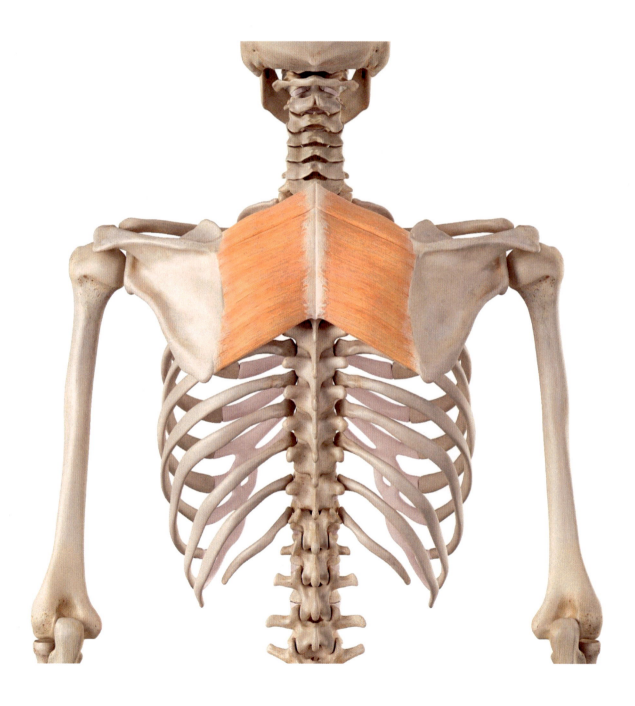

RHOMBOIDS: MAJOR & MINOR

Origin	Major: Nuchal ligament and spinous processes of C7-T1 / Minor: Spinous processes of T2-T5.
Insertion	Medial border of the scapula.
Action	Retracts and rotates the scapula downwards. Pull the scapula flat to the thorax.
Antagonist	Pectoralis major and minor.
Innervation	Dorsal scapular nerve C4-C5.
Blood Supply	Dorsal scapular artery.
Daily Use	Sitting or standing up straight (proud chest). Pulling something open.
Gym Use	Bent-over rows, single-arm rows, rear flys.

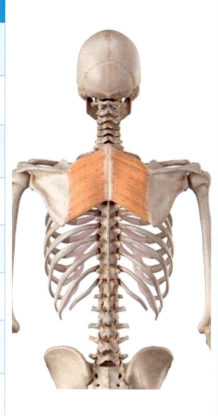

ROLLING THE RHOMBOIDS:

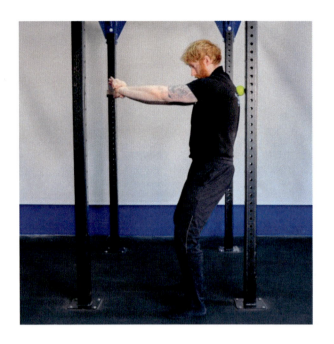

1. Standing: Place the massage ball on a wall, and while holding it with one hand, push your back into it to support the ball (this can be a little awkward).
2. Roll the ball into position – between your spine and shoulder blade.
3. Lying: Place the massage ball on the floor.
4. Lie onto the massage ball so that it is pushed into your rhomboids (a peanut ball can be used to target a section of both sides).
5. Knead the tissues for around 30-60 seconds.
6. Complete 1-2 times on each side.

RHOMBOID STRETCH:

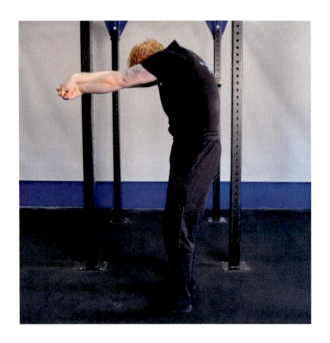

1. Stand upright in a hip-width stance.
2. Hold your arms to your front and internally rotate your shoulders to turn your palms outwards (thumbs down).
3. Cross your hands over each other and clasp your fingers together.
4. Push forward with your hands to protract your shoulders and as you do this, push your head down between your arms and round your upper back – push your arms forward and your back, back.
5. Hold for 30-60 seconds for a regular stretch, or 2 minutes if the musculature is very tense.
6. Complete 1-3 times on each side.

BAND RETRACTIONS:

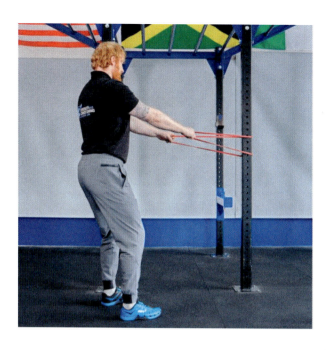

1. Use a low to medium-tension resistance band. The tension can be varied by standing closer or further away from the band attachment point.
2. Attach the band to something solid at abdominal/lower chest height. Facing the attachment point, grab each end of the band with a neutral grip.
3. Walk backwards to apply tension to the band.
4. Retract your shoulder to pull the band back.
5. Ensure you really concentrate on retracting your shoulders – mind-muscle connection.
6. Return to the starting position under control, allowing your shoulders to protract slightly.
7. Complete 2-3 sets of 10-20 reps.

BAND HORIZONTAL ROW:

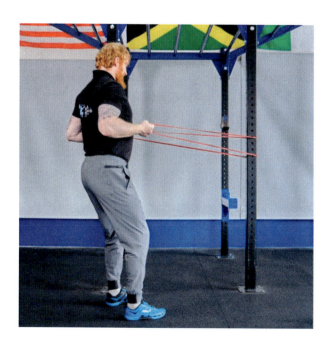

8. Use a low to medium-tension resistance band. The tension can be varied by standing closer or further away from the band attachment point.
9. Attach the band to something solid at abdominal/lower chest height. Facing the attachment point, grab each end of the band with a neutral grip.
10. Walk backwards to apply tension to the band.
11. Pull the band to your sides, ensuring you consciously engage your back muscles, rather than just pulling with your biceps (mind-muscle connection).
12. Ensure you really concentrate on retracting your shoulders.
13. Return to the starting position under control, allowing your shoulders to protract slightly.
14. Complete 2-3 sets of 10-20 reps.

BAND PULL APART:

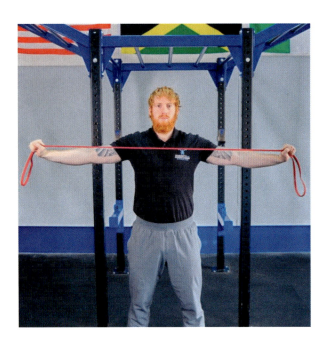

1. Use a low-tension band. The tension can be varied by taking a wider or narrower grip.
2. Take an overhand grip (palms facing down) on the band and place your arms out in front of you with your elbows straight. Grip the band at shoulder width if you can.
3. With your arms straight, pull your arms outwards so the band stretches and comes to your mid chest.
4. The band can also be pulled to your abdomen or forehead to vary the angle at which your shoulders are working.
5. Don't allow the band to jerk you back to the starting position. Keep it under control through the whole movement.
6. Complete 2-3 sets of 10-20 reps.

BAND STAR PATTERN PULL APART:

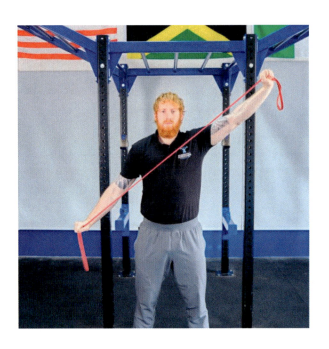

1. Start with the standard pull-apart to your mid-chest.
2. Pull your right hand downwards and your left arm upwards, so the band comes diagonally across your body.
3. Repeat this action but the opposite way around, right hand upwards and left hand downwards.
4. Repeat the standard pull apart to your upper chest to restart the cycle.
5. Complete 2-3 sets of 10-20 reps (each pull apart = 1 rep).

THE ABDOMINALS

Your anterior core musculature (abdominals) tends to get a lot of attention due to their importance aesthetically.

Although these muscles need to be strong, they can become excessively tense due to getting plenty of training without much stretching. This is often reinforced by prolonged sitting in a hunched posture that leaves them in a shortened position.

Both the rectus abdominis (6-pack muscles) and the obliques (musculature to the side of the 6-pack) all attach between your ribs and your pelvis, and any muscle mass that attaches to your pelvis can influence pelvic positioning and have a role in ailments such as low back pain.

Earlier, I discussed the importance of thoracic mobility and how to specifically target the area to ensure good posture and shoulder health. If your abdominal muscles are tight and pulling your rib cage closer to your pelvis, this will also affect your ability to extend your thoracic spine. So, this is an area that needs to be considered when trying to rectify thoracic mobility issues.

Tip: When sitting in a chair (car seat, etc), ensure your glutes are tucked right to the back of the seat. This will ensure you can sit up straight with ease – try it and you feel much taller in your seat.

THE TRANSVERSE ABDOMINIS

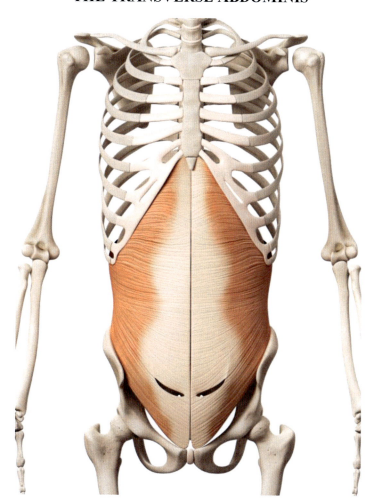

RECTUS ABDOMINIS

Origin	Anterior, inferior pubis.
Insertion	Cartilage of 5th to 7th ribs, and the base of the sternum.
Action	Flexes and laterally flexes the spine and posteriorly tilts the pelvis.
Antagonist	Erector spinae.
Innervation	Intercostal nerves T7-T11, subcostal nerve T12.
Blood Supply	Superior and inferior epigastric arteries.
Daily Use	Sitting up, coughing, sneezing, and defecating.
Gym Use	Sit-ups, leg raises, jack-knives. Work to maintain trunk/pelvic position during compound exercises.

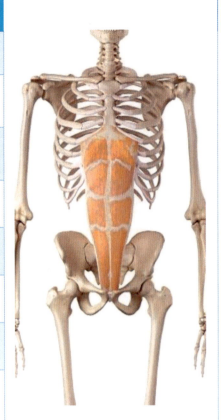

INTERNAL OBLIQUE

Origin	Iliac crest and thoracolumbar fascia.
Insertion	Lower 3 ribs, and the fascial connection to the linea alba.
Action	Rotates and laterally flexes and extends the spine (working on opposite sides).
Antagonist	Erector spinae, quadratus lumborum, and diaphragm.
Innervation	Thoracoabdominal T7-T11, Subcostal T12, Iliohypogastric L1, and Ilioinguinal nerve L1.
Blood Supply	Lower posterior intercostal and subcostal, and superior and inferior epigastric arteries.
Daily Use	Sitting up and reaching for an alarm clock, chopping wood, sweeping, and swinging a bat.
Gym Use	Band and cable rotations, rotational sit-ups, Russian twists, rotational throws.

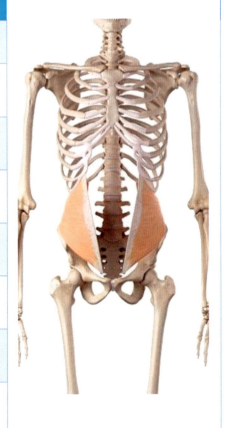

EXTERNAL OBLIQUE

Origin	Outer surface of ribs 6-12.
Insertion	Iliac crest, pubis, and fascial connection to the linea alba.
Action	Rotates and laterally flexes and extends the spine (working on opposite sides).
Antagonist	Erector spinae and quadratus lumborum.
Innervation	Thoracoabdominal nerves T7-11, subcostal nerve T12.
Blood Supply	Lower posterior intercostal, subcostal, and deep circumflex iliac arteries.
Daily Use	Sitting up and reaching for an alarm clock, chopping wood, sweeping, and swinging a bat.
Gym Use	Band and cable rotations, rotational sit-ups, Russian twists, rotational throws.

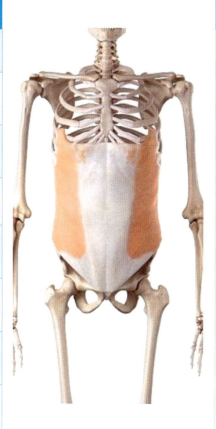

ROLLING THE ABDOMINALS:

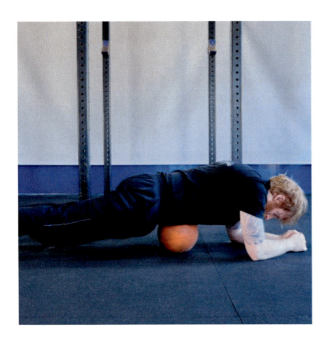

1. Place a medicine ball on the floor – softer balls work well.
2. Lie onto the ball and apply pressure to the abdominals – caution should be practiced due to the fact the abdominal wall provides less protection to the viscera (internal organs) compared to the lower back muscles.
3. Knead the tissues for around 30-60 seconds.
4. Complete 1-2 times.
5. You can also contract the abdominals into the ball before relaxing onto the ball – complete 3-5 times.

COBRA ABDOMINAL STRETCH:

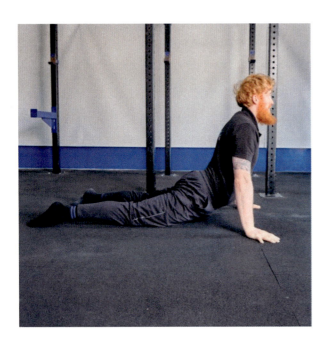

1. Lie on your stomach.
2. While keeping your hips on the floor, use your forearms or hands to raise your torso up.
3. You will be hyperextending through your spine as you rise, so take care.
4. To regress the stretch, come up onto your forearms rather than your hands.
5. To vary the stretch to work your obliques, simply lean to one side. Explore the positions to find the optimal stretch.
6. Hold for 30-60 seconds, or 2 minutes if the musculature is very tense.
7. Complete 1-3 times.

STANDING ABDOMINAL STRETCH:

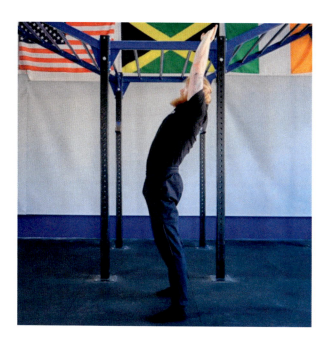

1. Stand up straight in a shoulder-width or slightly wider stance.
2. Place one hand over the other and take your arms overhead.
3. Reach backwards and allow your hips and lower spine to hyperextend.
4. Hold for 30-60 seconds – this position can restrict your breathing so it is unlikely that it will be held for longer too long (regulate your breathing).
5. Complete 1-3 times.

DEAD BUG:

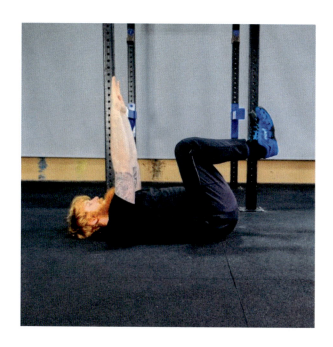

1. Lie on your back with your head flat on the floor.
2. Tilt your pelvis to flatten your lower back to the floor. Ensure you maintain this position throughout the exercise.
3. Extend your arms up to the front, with your palms facing forward.
4. Raise your feet up, bending your knees and hips at 90 degrees (this is your starting position).
5. Slowly extend your right leg to a point where your heel is just off the floor.
6. At the same time, flex your left arm to take it overhead, bringing it to a point where your hand is just off the floor.
7. Slowly return your leg and arm back to the starting position and proceed with the opposite sides.
8. Perform 3-5 sets of 5-10 reps on each side.

PALLOF PRESS/ISO HOLD:

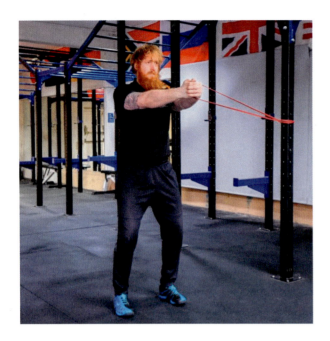

1. Use a low-tension resistance band. The tension can be varied by standing closer to, or further away from the band attachment point if required.
2. Attach the band to something solid at chest height, looping the band through itself.
3. Grab the band with both hands and stand side-on to the attachment point, holding your hands at your chest.
4. Sidestep away from the attachment point to add tension to the band.
5. Ensure that your feet, hips and shoulders are forward facing. Don't counter the band tension by turning away from the attachment point.
6. For an isometric hold, press the band out and hold it for 30-40 seconds.
7. If performing the pallof press, engage your core and press the band to your front, holding it for 2-5 seconds, before returning it to the starting position and proceeding with successive reps.
8. Complete 2-3 sets of 30-40 seconds or 5-15 reps on each side.

FRONT PLANK:

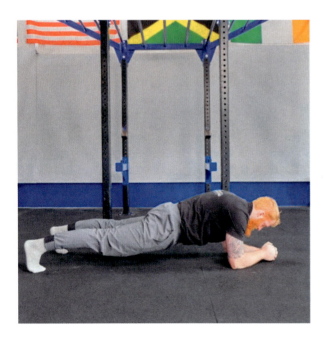

1. Kneel on the floor and clasp your hands together so that your forearms are at a 45-degree angle.
2. Place your forearms onto the floor just as you would during a standard front plank. To increase the intensity, place your arms further forward, so that your elbows sit in front of your shoulders.
3. Step back with your left then right foot at hip to shoulder width. You can also have your legs together and maximally engage your adductors (inner thighs).
4. Maximally contract your glutes and abs, which will tilt your pelvis back slightly.
5. Maximally contract your quads and core musculature. Pull back with your forearms (as if you are pulling your elbows towards your toes) to increase your core engagement.
6. Complete 3-5 sets of 30-60 seconds.

SIDE PLANK:

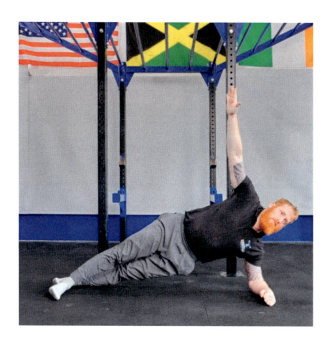

1. Lie on your right-hand side and place your right forearm onto the floor, perpendicular to your body.
2. Placing your left foot on the front of your right foot helps to keep your hips in a balanced position and allows you to easily transition between front and side plank variations.
3. Raise your hips so there is no side bending of your spine and so that your lower legs are raised off the floor.
4. Engage your glutes, so your hips are extended. Having slightly bent hips is a common fault.
5. Maximally brace your core musculature, as you would during an front plank.
6. Either keep your left arm flat to your body or raise it to the sky.
7. Complete 2-3 sets of 30-60 seconds on each side.

CURL-UP:

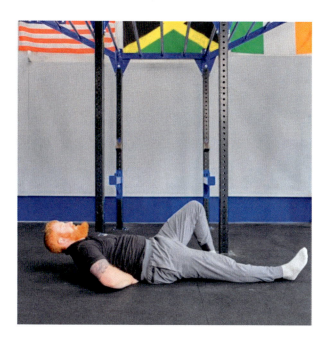

1. Lie down with your head flat on the floor.
2. Bend your left leg, bringing your heel up towards your glutes, while keeping your right leg extended.
3. Bend your elbows and place your hands under your lower back. This ensures you maintain a neutral spine throughout the movement. Keeping your elbows raised off the floor throughout the movement makes it harder.
4. Slowly raise your head and shoulders up a few inches and maximally contract your abs for 10 seconds before slowly returning to the starting position.
5. Try not to roll your chin towards your chest. Keep your chin retracted as you raise your shoulders and head up.
6. Complete 2-3 sets of 5 reps with 10 second pauses at the top.

SIT-UP:

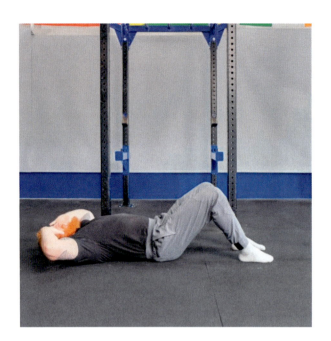

7. Lie down with your head flat on the floor.
8. Bend your legs so your feet are flat on the floor (you can use a foot anchor – something to hold your feet down).
9. Cross your arms across your chest or hold your fingers against your temples.
10. Engage your abdominals to raise your torso up.
11. You can perform half-sit ups (crunches) or raise up all the way (more hip flexor engagement).
12. You can also rotate at the top of the sit-up.
13. Complete 2-3 sets of 10-20 reps.

THE RIBCAGE

The upper spine is made up of 12 thoracic vertebrae, and each of these 12 vertebrae has a rib on either side, making a total of 24 ribs (12 pairs).

The first seven ribs (from the top down) insert directly onto the sternum (breastbone) and are referred to as true/fixed ribs. The next 5 are referred to as false ribs, the first 3 of these connect to the sternum indirectly via the costal cartilages and the final 2 are referred to as floating ribs because they are only attached to the vertebrae.

The ribcage protects internal organs and is involved in respiration.

The ribcage provides attachment sites for several key muscles, such as the serratus anterior.

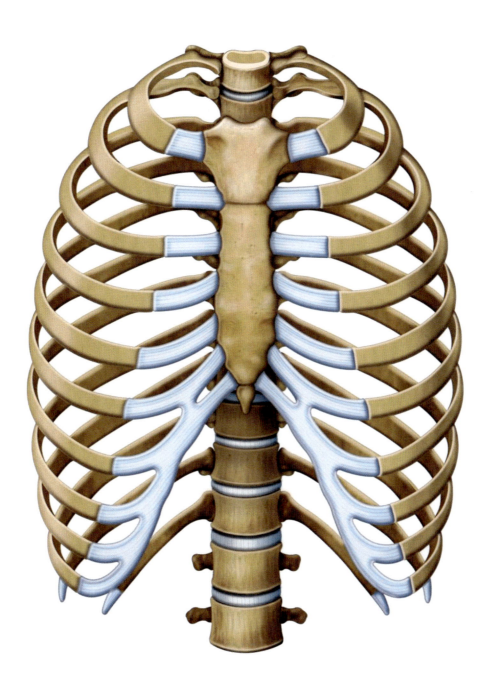

THE SERRATUS ANTERIOR

The serratus anterior is a muscle that attaches between your shoulder blade's inner surface and your ribcage.

The serratus anterior works to protract and rotate the shoulder blades upwards (upward rotation) – upward rotation is extremely important when pressing overhead.

Note: We also have serratus posterior muscles (inferior and superior), which work as respiratory muscles, with the inferior working to pull the lower ribs down, and the superior working to elevate the second to the fifth rib.

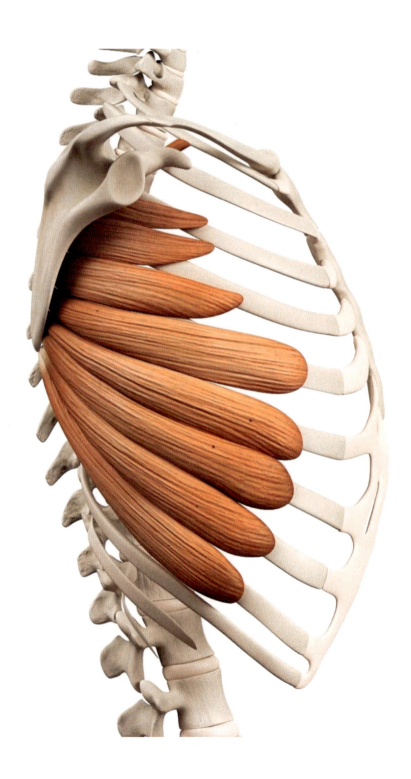

SERRATUS ANTERIOR	
Origin	Surface of upper 8 or 9 ribs.
Insertion	Anterior surface of medial border of scapula.
Action	Protracts the scapula.
Antagonist	Rhomboids and lower trapezius.
Innervation	Long thoracic nerve C5-C7.
Blood Supply	Superior and lateral thoracic arteries, and thoracodorsal artery branches.
Daily Use	Reaching for a door handle, taking your arms overhead, pointing at something, striking.
Gym Use	Serratus wall slides, push-ups, pullovers.

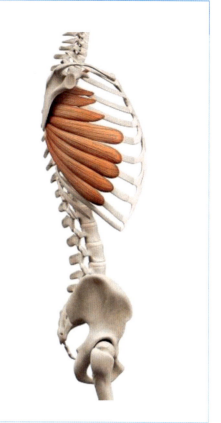

ROLLING THE SERRATUS ANTERIOR:

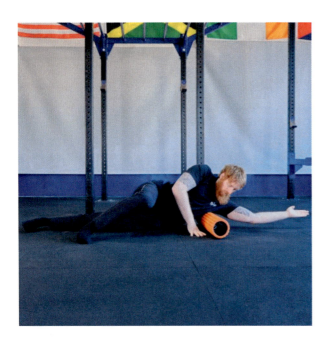

1. Sit down on the floor with the foam roller to your left side.
2. Raise your left arm up and lie down on your side, with the foam roller placed onto the serratus anterior (slightly forward of the lats onto the ribcage).
3. Slowly roll up and down the muscle mass for 30-60 seconds.
4. Repeat on the opposite side.
5. Complete 1-2 times on each side.

SERRATUS ANTERIOR STRETCH:

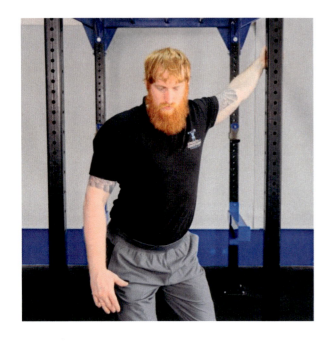

1. Stand up and reach high to grab a solid structure.
2. Sit back with your hips and rotate your chest away from the solid structure to increase the stretch on your serratus anterior.
3. Hold the stretch for 30-60 seconds, or 2 minutes if the musculature is very tense.
4. Complete 1-3 times on each side.

SCAPULA PUSH-UPS:

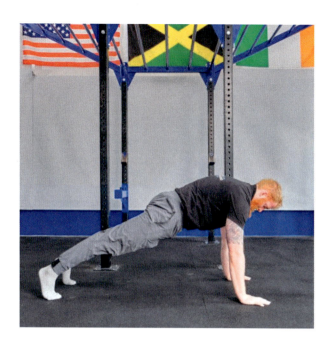

1. Get into a high plank position – the top of a push-up.
2. While keeping your arms straight, push your hands into the floor and aim to push your mid-upper back up towards the ceiling.
3. Your shoulder blades should abduct (move away from your spine) and your mid-upper back should round.
4. Perform 2-3 sets of 5-15 reps.

SERRATUS WALL SLIDES:

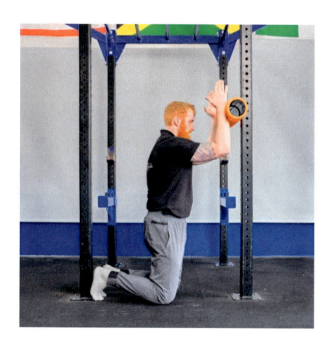

1. Place the roller against a wall.
2. Facing the wall/foam roller, bend your elbows to 90 degrees and place your forearms on the roller, with the roller just below your wrists.
3. Drive your forearms into the roller as if you are pushing yourself away, extending your shoulders and engaging the serratus.
4. Keep your head back and roll the roller up so that your shoulders flex and your elbows start to extend.
5. Feel your serratus engage and roll until the roller meets your elbow. Imagine the bottom of your shoulder blades rotating outwards and upwards towards your armpit.
6. Relax as you roll back down to the starting position.
7. Complete 2-4 sets of 5-10 reps.

THE PECTORALS

The pectorals (pecs) are the muscles of the chest and consist of the pectoralis major (largest) and the pectoralis minor (smallest).

The pec muscles are involved in pushing actions as they bring the arms forward.

Due to the popularity of pushing exercises in the gym, and the fact that much of our daily activities involve reaching forward or having our hands to the front (often slouching), the pecs can become tense and round the shoulders.

If the pecs are tense, it can restrict your ability to take your arms overhead, specifically during exercises such as the overhead squat.

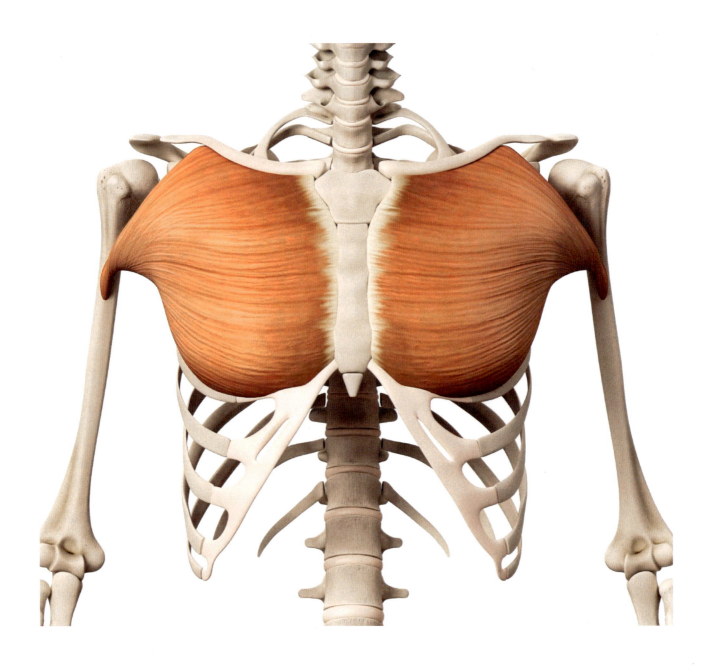

PECTORALIS MAJOR	
Origin	Clavicle and sternum.
Insertion	Humerus.
Action	Flexes, horizontally flexes, adducts and internally rotates the shoulder.
Antagonist	Deltoid.
Innervation	Lateral and medial pectoral nerves C5-T1.
Blood Supply	Pectoral branch of the thoracoacromial artery.
Daily Use	Pushing a door open, sawing a piece of wood.
Gym Use	Push-up, bench press, dumbbells fly.

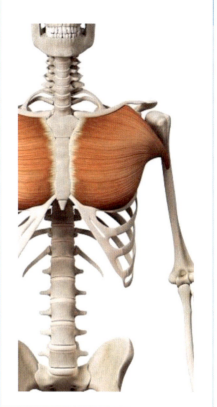

PECTORALIS MINOR	
Origin	Anterior surface of 3rd - 5th ribs.
Insertion	Coracoid process of scapula.
Action	Depresses and protracts the scapula.
Antagonist	Rhomboids and lower trapezius.
Innervation	Lateral and medial pectoral nerves C5-T1.
Blood Supply	Pectoral branch of the thoracoacromial artery.
Daily Use	Reaching for a door handle, reaching into your trouser pocket.
Gym Use	Push-up, bench press, dumbbells fly.

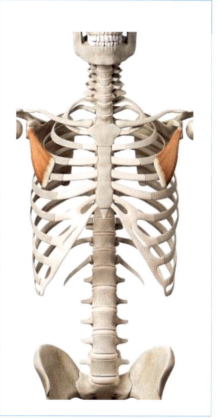

ROLLING THE PECTORALS:

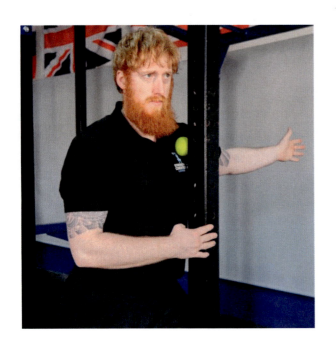

1. Place a massage ball onto a post at chest height.
2. Push your chest into the ball, just to the side of your armpit to target the pec minor.
3. Knead the tissues for 30-60 seconds.
4. You can flex your shoulder at 90 degrees and slowly horizontally flex and extend the shoulder to maximize the effectiveness of the release – perform 5-10 horizontal flexions and extensions.
5. Complete 1-2 times on each side.

CHAIR PECTORAL RELEASE:

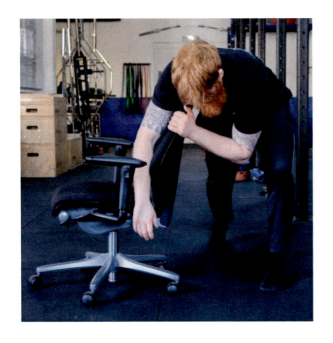

1. Stand behind a chair.
2. Place your right arm over the back of the chair.
3. Push the soft tissue between your chest and your arm into the top of the chair (just in from your armpit).
4. Knead the tissues for 30-60 seconds.
5. Repeat on the opposite side.
6. Complete 1-2 times on each side.

BARBELL PECTORAL RELEASE:

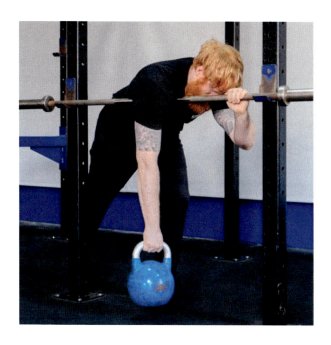

1. Set a barbell up on a rack at hip height.
2. Place your right arm over the barbell.
3. Drive the soft tissue between your chest and your arm into the barbell (just in from your armpit).
4. A weight (dumbbell/kettlebell) can be used to increase the pressure placed on the soft tissues.
5. Slowly move your arm forward and back and in small circles (with or without weight).
6. Knead the tissues for 30-60 seconds.
7. Complete 1-2 times on each side.

STANDING PECTORAL STRETCH:

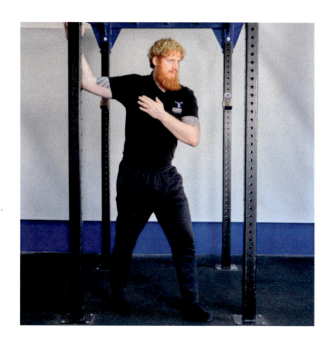

1. Raise your hand up with your elbow bent at 90 degrees.
2. Place your forearm along the edge of the door frame/wall/post and turn your body away from your arm.
3. Hold for 30-60 seconds for a regular stretch or 2 minutes if the musculature is very tense.
4. Complete 1-3 times.

SEATED PECTORAL STRETCH:

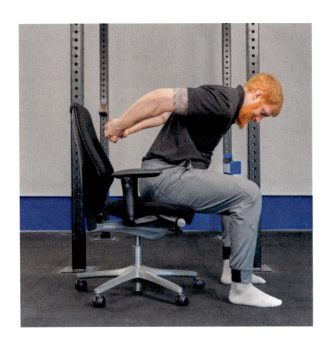

1. Sit on the front edge of your chair.
2. Clasp your hands together behind your back.
3. Lean forward and raise your hands up behind you.
4. Hold for 30-60 seconds for a regular stretch, or 2 minutes if the musculature is very tense.
5. Complete 1-3 times.

LYING PECTORAL STRETCH:

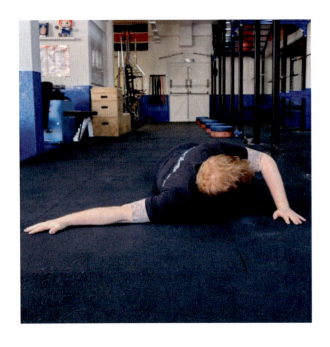

1. Lie on your front with your arms stretched out to your sides at shoulder height.
2. Lean over onto one side to stretch the pec and shoulder of that side.
3. Hold for 30-60 seconds for a regular stretch, or 2 minutes if the musculature is very tense.
4. Complete 1-3 times.

BAND PECTORAL STRETCH:

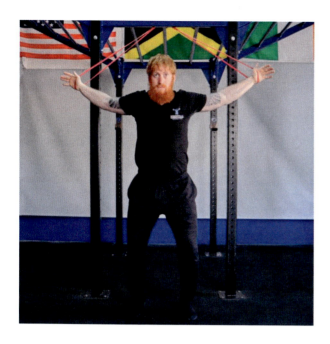

1. Attach a low-tension band to a solid structure – the height can be modified to create different stretches.
2. Hold each end of the band and turn your back to the band attachment point.
3. Raise your arms up to the sides (palms forward) and step forward to apply tension to the band and increase the stretch.
4. You can move the position of your arms to target different areas of the pecs and shoulders.
5. Ensure you fully support the position with your legs (don't lean too far into the stretch) – you shouldn't be at risk of falling.
6. Hold for 30-60 seconds for a regular stretch, or 2 minutes if the musculature is very tense.
7. Complete 1-3 times.

PARTNER PECTORAL PNF:

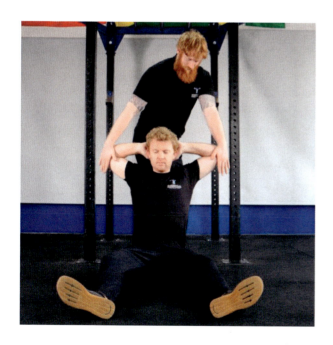

1. Have the client sit on the floor and place their hands behind their head.
2. Stand behind the client and place the outer side of your leg against their back to support the position.
3. Pull back on their elbows to reach the barrier position.
4. Hold the stretch for 10-15 seconds before releasing it slightly and instructing the client to push their arms into your hands.
5. Instruct the client to push with 50-60% intensity for 6-8 seconds.
6. Instruct the client to stop contracting and allow 1-2 seconds for the muscle to relax fully. During this time, instruct the client to take a deep breath in.
7. Instruct the client to exhale slowly, and as they do, pull the arms into the next barrier position and hold for 10-15 seconds.
8. Repeat the previous steps 2-3 times and hold the final position for 20-30+ seconds.
9. Complete the stretch on both sides.

SOLO PECTORAL PNF:

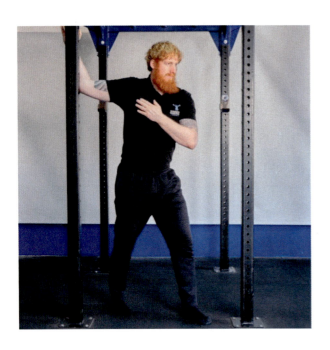

1. Stand and raise your hand up with your elbow bent at 90 degrees.
2. Place your forearm along the edge of the door frame/wall/post and turn your body away from your arm to reach the barrier position.
3. Hold the stretch for 10-15 seconds before releasing it slightly and pushing your forearm into the structure – 50-60% intensity for 6-8 seconds.
4. Stop contracting, take a deep breath in, and allow 1-2 seconds for the muscle to relax fully.
5. Exhale slowly and turn your body away from your arm to reach the next barrier position and hold for 10-15 seconds.
6. Repeat the previous steps 2-3 times and hold the final position for 20-30+ seconds.
7. Complete the stretch on both sides.

BAND FLY:

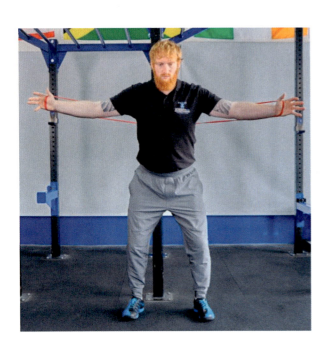

1. Loop a low-tension band around the back of a solid structure at around shoulder height.
2. Grab each end of the band and turn around – face away from the attachment point.
3. Walk forward to apply tension to the band and bring your arms up to around shoulder height with slightly bent elbows.
4. The exercise can be performed with an upright or a slightly bent over posture.
5. Squeeze the chest to horizontally adduct your arms, bringing your hands together or crossing them over each other to the front.
6. Perform 2-3 sets of 10 reps.

SINGLE-ARM BAND FLY:

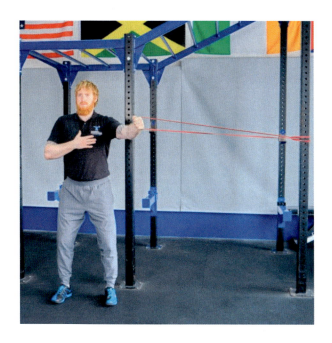

1. Loop a low-tension band around the back of a solid structure or through itself around the post at around shoulder height.
2. Grab the band with one hand and stand side onto the attachment point.
3. Walk away from the attachment point to apply tension to the band and bring arm up to around shoulder height with a slightly bent elbow.
4. Squeeze the chest to horizontally adduct your arms, bringing your hands together or crossing them over each other to the front.
5. Perform 2-3 sets of 10 reps on each side.

DUMBBELL FLY:

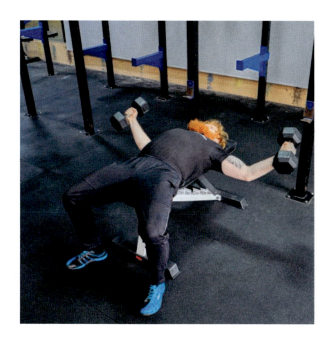

1. Grab a dumbbell in each hand and lie on a bench.
2. Press the dumbbells and bring them together with your palms facing each other.
3. Bend your elbows slightly – retain this elbow bend throughout the entire range of motion.
4. Open your arms to lower the dumbbells until your upper arms are in line or slightly below your torso.
5. Contact your chest muscles to bring the weight back together.
6. Perform 2-3 sets of 10 reps.

THE SHOULDERS

The shoulder joint is made up between the glenoid fossa on the scapula (socket) and the humeral head (ball), which is the top of the humerus (upper arm bone).

The shoulder girdle is made up between the scapula and the clavicle (collar bone). The scapular attaches to the clavicle via the acromion process, which creates the acromioclavicular (AC) joint.

The shoulders are ball and socket joints and have the greatest ROM of any joint in the body.

The muscles that we are looking at in this section are the rotator cuff and the deltoid.

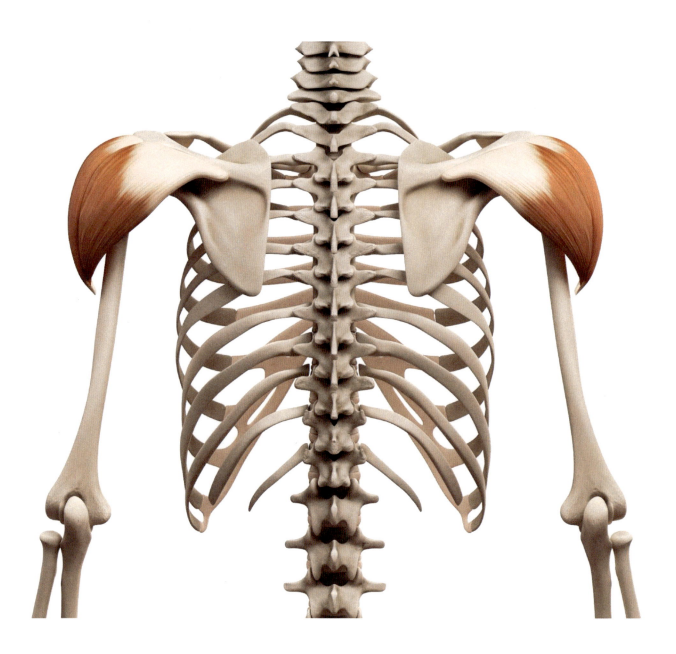

THE ROTATOR CUFF

The rotator cuff is made up of four muscles that originate on the scapular and insert onto the humeral head. Therefore, they specifically work to stabilize the shoulder joint.

The attachment points are what define these muscles as rotator cuff. For example, some may ask why the teres minor is a rotator cuff, but the teres major is not, and this is because the teres major inserts lower on the humerus and therefore, primarily works to assist the latissimus dorsi in shoulder extension and adduction rather than specifically working to stabilize the joint. However, it should be noted that any muscle close to a joint, plays some role in supporting it.

The four rotator cuff:

- Supraspinatus / Infraspinatus / Teres Minor / Subscapularis.

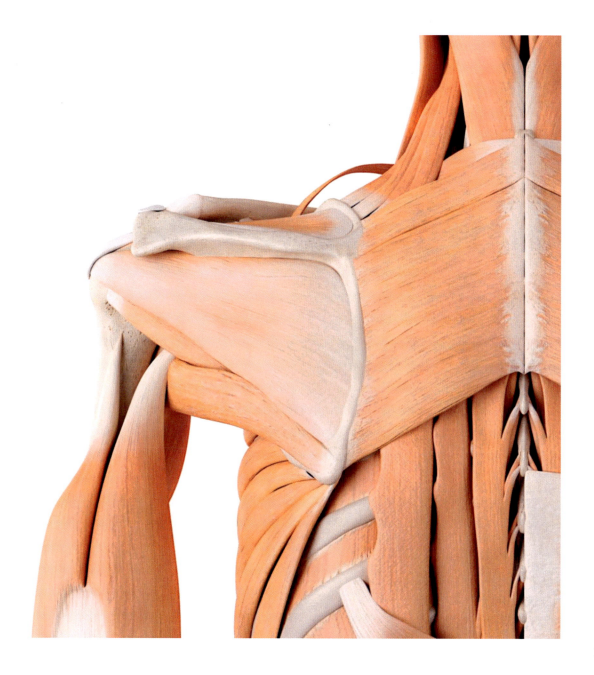

SUPRASPINATUS	
Origin	Superior surface of scapula (above spine of scapula).
Insertion	Upper humerus.
Action	Stabilizes and abducts the shoulder.
Antagonist	Latissimus dorsi and pectoralis major.
Innervation	Suprascapular nerve C5-C6.
Blood Supply	Suprascapular artery.
Daily Use	Bringing your arm out to the side.
Gym Use	Lateral raises, throwing.

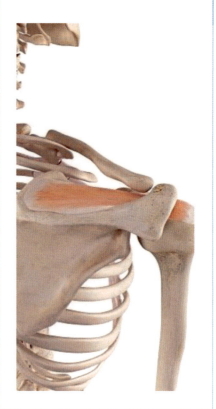

INFRASPINATUS	
Origin	Posterior surface of scapula (below spine of scapula).
Insertion	Upper humerus.
Action	Stabilizes and externally rotates the shoulder.
Antagonist	Subscapularis.
Innervation	Suprascapular nerve C5-C6.
Blood Supply	Suprascapular and circumflex scapular arteries.
Daily Use	Fanning your face with your hand, shaking a can.
Gym Use	Band external rotations, face pulls.

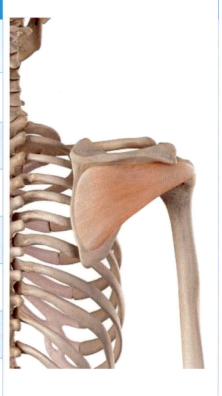

TERES MINOR	
Origin	Lateral border of the scapula.
Insertion	Upper humerus.
Action	Stabilizes and externally rotates the shoulder.
Antagonist	Subscapularis.
Innervation	Axillary nerve C5-C6
Blood Supply	Suprascapular, and dorsal scapular artery
Daily Use	Fanning your face with your hand, shaking a can.
Gym Use	Band external rotations, face pulls.

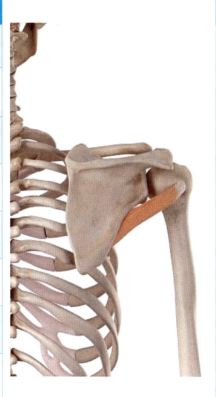

SUBSCAPULARIS	
Origin	Anterior surface of the Scapula.
Insertion	Upper humerus.
Action	Stabilizes and internally rotates the shoulder.
Antagonist	Infraspinatus and teres minor.
Innervation	Upper and lower subscapular nerves C5-C6.
Blood Supply	Subscapular, axillary, and subscapular arteries.
Daily Use	Scratching your lower back.
Gym Use	Band internal rotations.

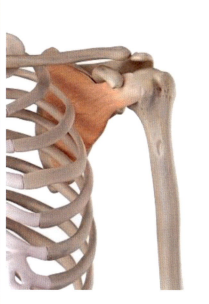

ROLLING THE EXTERNAL ROTATORS:

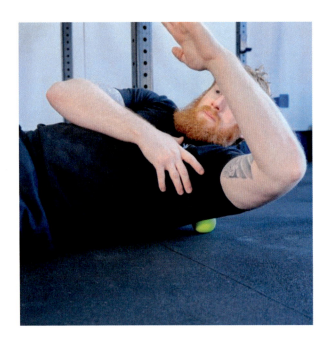

1. Sit down onto the floor and place a massage ball onto the floor.
2. Lie onto the ball with, anywhere from your shoulder blade to your shoulder – have your elbow bent at 90 degrees.
3. Knead the tissues for 30-60 seconds.
4. You can internally and externally rotate your shoulder to maximize the effectiveness of the release – perform 5-10 internal and external rotations.
5. Complete 1-2 times on each side.

DOWEL EXTERNAL ROTATOR STRETCH:

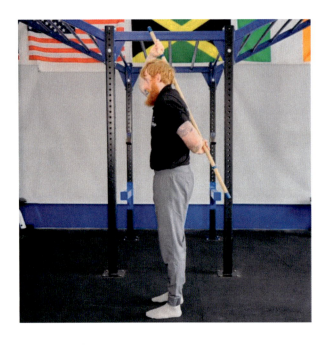

1. Take a dowel in your left hand and bring your left hand behind your back so the dowel is running up your back and over your head.
2. Take your right hand overhead and grab the dowel.
3. Gently pull the dowel forward with your right hand, either over your right or left shoulder (try both and see which one feels best).
4. Hold for 30-60 seconds for a regular stretch, or 2 minutes if the musculature is very tense.
5. Complete 1-3 times on each side.

DOWEL INTERNAL ROTATOR STRETCH:

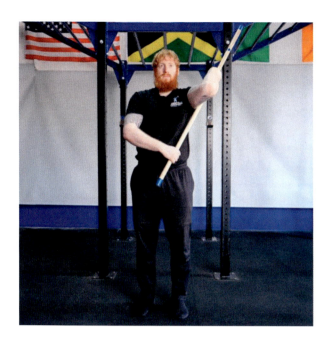

1. Grab a dowel in your left hand.
2. Bend your elbow fully and externally rotate your shoulder. This will bring the dowel onto the outer side of your left arm.
3. Bring your right arm under your left arm and grab the dowel.
4. Gently pull on the dowel to apply the stretch.
5. Hold for 30-60 seconds for a regular stretch, or 2 minutes if the musculature is very tense.
6. Complete 1-3 times on each side.

BACK SCRATCH STRETCH:

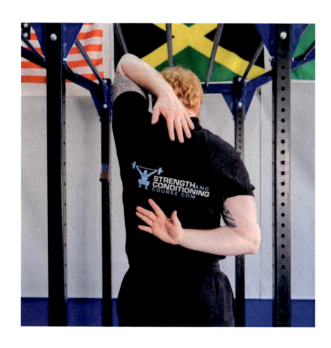

1. Stand up straight and place one hand over your shoulder and behind your head (palm facing your back and fingers down).
2. Place your other arm behind your lower back (palm facing outward and fingers upward).
3. Push the arms towards each other to increase the stretch. However, caution should be practiced not to place maladaptive stress on the shoulder joints.
4. A towel or band can be used to assist the stretch, either pulling down to increase the stretch on the top arm or pulling up to increase the stretch on the bottom arm.
5. Hold for 30-60 seconds for a regular stretch, or 2 minutes if the musculature is very tense.
6. Complete 1-3 times on each side.

BAND BULLY STRETCH:

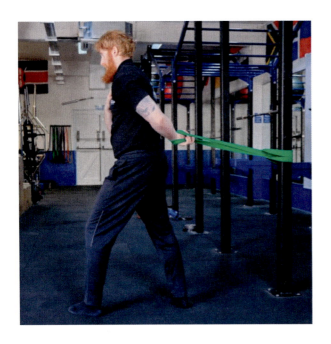

1. Attach a medium to high-tension band to a solid structure.
2. Grab the end of the band with one arm.
3. Turn away from to bring your hand behind your back.
4. Step away from the band to apply tension to it and increase the stretch.
5. Caution should be practiced to ensure you are not placing maladaptive stress to the shoulder joint.
6. Hold for 30-60 seconds for a regular stretch, or 2 minutes if the musculature is very tense.
7. Complete 1-3 times on each side.

BAND INTERNAL ROTATION:

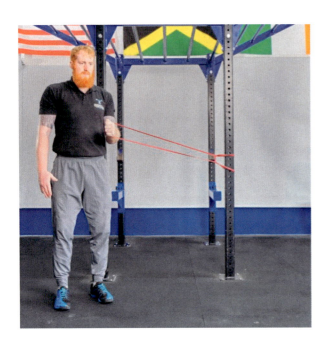

1. Attach a low-tension band to a solid structure. You can increase tension by standing further from the attachment point.
2. Grab the band with your right hand and turn side on so that your right shoulder is closest to the attachment point.
3. Stand with good posture, bend your right elbow to 90 degrees and keep it tucked into your side.
4. Pull the band across your body while internally rotating your right shoulder. Ensure your body stays forward facing and your right elbow remains tucked into your side.
5. Once you have reached the limit of your range of motion with your elbow tucked in, slowly return to the starting position.
6. Complete 2-3 sets of 10-15 reps on each side.

BAND EXTERNAL ROTATION:

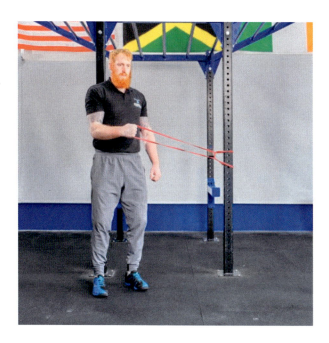

1. Attach a low-tension band to a solid structure. You can increase tension by standing further from the attachment point.
2. Grab the band with your right hand and turn side on so that your right shoulder is closest to the attachment point.
3. Stand with good posture, bend your right elbow to 90 degrees and keep it tucked into your side.
4. Pull the band across your body while internally rotating your right shoulder. Ensure your body stays forward facing and your right elbow remains tucked into your side.
5. Once you have reached the limit of your range of motion with your elbow tucked in, slowly return to the starting position.
6. If your elbow comes away from your side, your large shoulder muscle (delt) will take over, so it's important to hold it close.
7. Complete 2-3 sets of 10-15 reps on each side.

BAND FACE PULL:

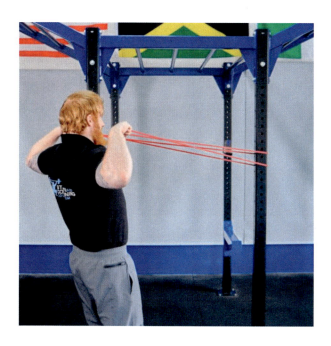

1. Use a low-tension resistance band. You can alter the tension by standing closer or further away from the band attachment point.
2. Attach the band to something solid at chest height.
3. Facing the attachment point, grab the band with an overhand grip. Or you can grab the band with just your fingers, rather than a full grip, to help encourage the upper back to work as the primary mover rather than the biceps.
4. Step backwards to apply tension to the band.
5. Keep your chin back.
6. Pull backwards and slightly upward to bring yourself into a double bicep pose position.
7. Ensure you consciously engage your upper back and rear delts rather than just pulling with your biceps. Visualize the muscle you are working to increase its engagement and build mind-muscle connection.
8. Return to the starting position under control, allowing your shoulders to extend slightly.
9. Complete 2-3 sets of 10-20 reps.

THE DELTOIDS

The deltoids are the coconut shaped muscle at the top of the arms.

The deltoids are made up of 3 distinct fibres:

- Anterior (Clavicular) Fibres.

- Medial/Middle (Acromion) Fibres.

- Posterior (Scapula) Fibres.

The fibres to the front (anterior) will work pressing actions to the front and overhead and horizontal flexion.

The fibres in the middle (medial) work abduction and pressing overhead, and the fibres to the rear (posterior) will work during pulling actions and horizontal extension.

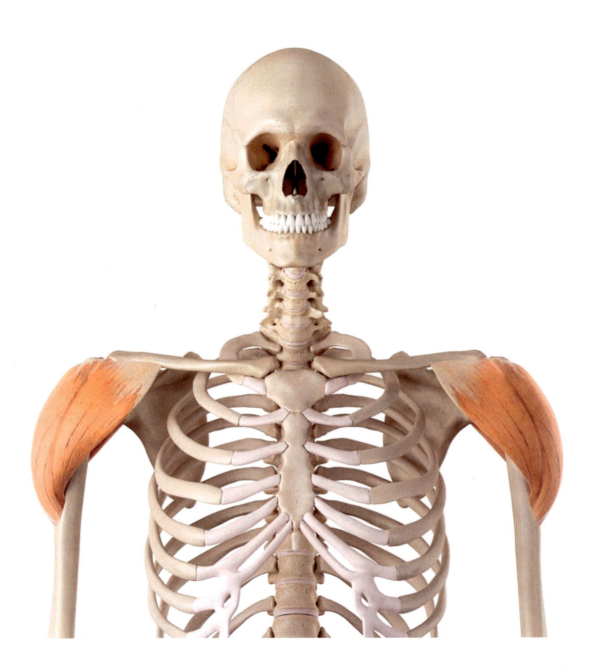

DELTOID	
Origin	Clavicle and upper scapula.
Insertion	Upper humerus.
Action	Abducts, flexes, extends, horizontally flexes and extends, and rotates the shoulder.
Antagonist	Latissimus dorsi.
Innervation	Axillary nerve C5-C6.
Blood Supply	Thoracoacromial artery, anterior and posterior humeral circumflex artery.
Daily Use	Most movements that involve the arms, lifting a drink to your mouth.
Gym Use	Lateral raises, bench press, bent-over rows.

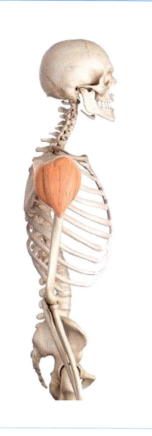

ROLLING THE DELTOIDS:

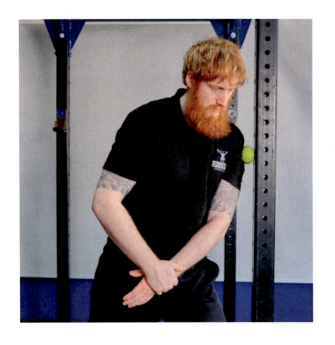

1. Place a massage ball against a wall/post and support it with one hand.
2. Lean into the ball with your shoulder.
3. Knead the tissues for around 30-60 seconds.
4. Complete 1-2 times on each side.

BARBELL ROLLING THE DELTOIDS:

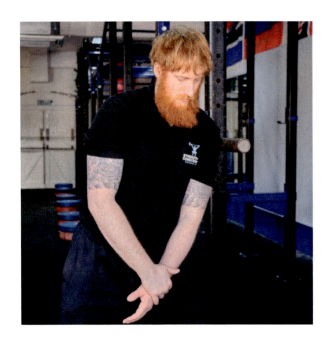

1. Set a barbell up on the rack at upper chest height
2. Stand in front of the rack so when you push your deltoid into the barbell, it pushes it back into the rack/J-cup (as pictured).
3. Lean into the sleeve of the barbell with your deltoid.
4. Slowly roll up and down (knead) the muscle for 30-60 seconds.
5. Complete 1-2 times on each side.

MEDIAL-POSTERIOR DELTOID STRETCH:

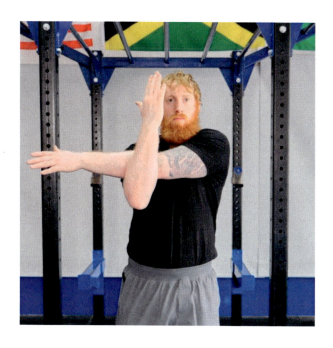

1. Bring your one arm across your upper chest.
2. Bring your other arm up and place it either above or below your elbow – having it below the elbow will allow for a greater stretch
3. Pull back on the straight arm to increase the stretch.
4. Hold for 30-60 seconds for a regular stretch, or 2 minutes if the musculature is very tense.
5. Complete 1-3 times on each side.

ANTERIOR DELTOID STRETCH:

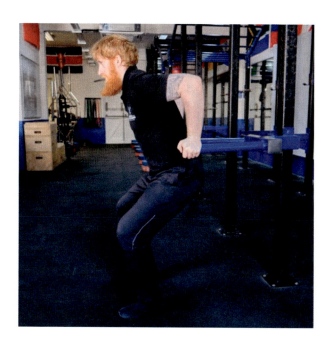

1. Stand with your back to the raised surface (kitchen surface, windowsill, etc).
2. Bring your elbows back so you can place your palms onto the raised surface.
3. Drop your body down under control to apply a stretch.
4. Hold for 30-60 seconds for a regular stretch, or 2 minutes if the musculature is very tense.
5. Complete 1-3 times.

BAND FRONT TO BACKS:

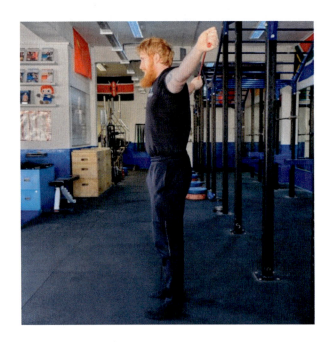

1. Grab a red band with a wide overhand grip. The wider your arms, the easier it is to take the band overhead and down towards your glutes.
2. The band gives you the freedom to widen your grip as you pass it overhead. Your grip should be wide enough so that you aren't forced to aggressively stretch the band out as you perform the movement, as this can cause you to shrug your shoulders, engaging musculature rather than promoting mobility.
3. Start with the band at your hips and while maintaining straight arms throughout, pass it overhead until it reaches your glutes, or the range of motion you can achieve.
4. Complete 2-3 sets of 5-10 reps.

LATERAL RAISE:

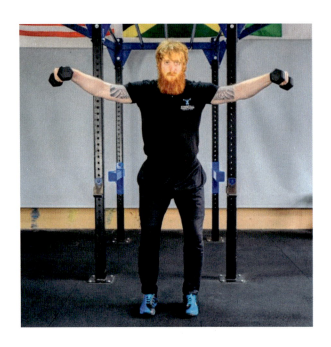

1. Hold a dumbbell in each hand.
2. Stand in a whip-width stance.
3. Leaning forward slightly will help to increase the engagement of the posterior deltoids.
4. Engage your delts and raise your arms up to your sides.
5. Bring the dumbbells up in line with your shoulders while maintaining a slight bend in your elbows.
6. Complete 2-3 sets of 10-15 reps.

YWT:

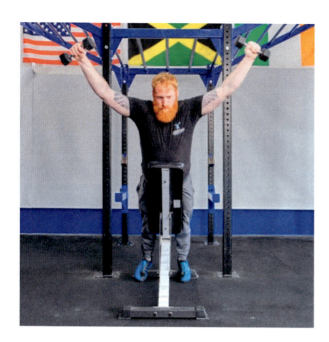

1. Grab a light dumbbell in each hand.
2. Lie on your front on an inclines bench.
3. Allow your arms to hang down to your front.
4. Raise your arms up above your head in a "Y" position.
5. Lower your arms back to the starting position.
6. Raise your arms up into a "W" position – biceps pose.
7. Lower your arms back to the starting position (elbows bent at 90 degrees).
8. Raise your arms up into a "T" position – arms out to your sides (straight arms).
9. Lower your arms back to the starting position.
10. Repeat the cycle.
11. Complete 2-3 sets of 3-5 cycles.

THE UPPER ARMS

The upper arms are made up between the biceps and the triceps. The biceps flex the elbow, and the triceps extend the elbow.

The primary biceps muscle is known as the biceps brachii and has two heads, meaning it has two origins.

Other biceps muscles include:

- Brachialis.

- Brachioradialis.

- Coracobrachialis.

The primary triceps muscle is known as the triceps brachii and has three heads (three origins).

Another muscle that assists in elbow extension is the anconeus.

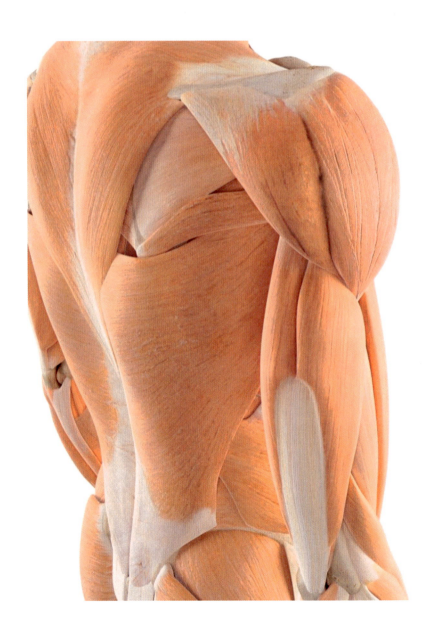

THE BICEPS

The biceps are the muscle on the front of the arm and flex our elbows. Therefore, whenever we hold an object in our hands with a bent elbow, our biceps are contracting.

The biceps brachii also works to flex the shoulder because they originate on the shoulder blade.

The biceps tend to get a lot of attention in the gym (especially by males). Not only are they individually trained, but they are also worked whenever we train pulling movements – deadlift, rows, pull-ups, etc.

Despite all this work on the biceps, the muscle group rarely gets much attention when to release techniques and stretches, which can lead them to become tense.

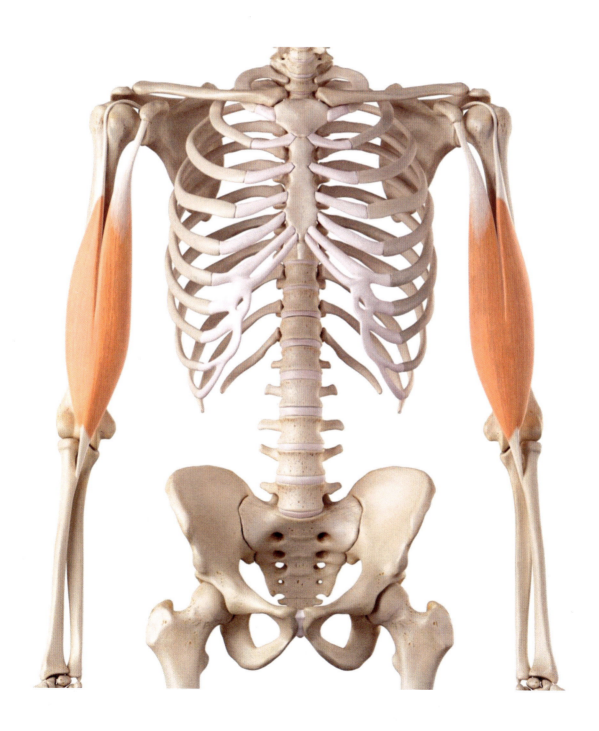

BICEPS BRACHII	
Origin	Anterior surface of the Scapula.
Insertion	Upper radius.
Action	Flexes the elbow and shoulder and supinates the forearm.
Antagonist	Triceps brachii.
Innervation	Musculocutaneous nerve C5–C6.
Blood Supply	Brachial artery.
Daily Use	Picking something up, using a screwdriver.
Gym Use	Biceps curls, rows, throws, strikes.

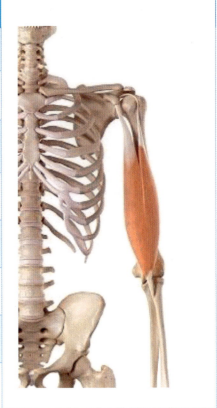

BRACHIALIS	
Origin	Front surface of the humerus.
Insertion	Upper ulna.
Action	Flexes the elbow.
Antagonist	Triceps brachii.
Innervation	Musculocutaneous nerve C5-C6, and radial nerve C7.
Blood Supply	Brachial, and radial recurrent arteries.
Daily Use	Picking something up, using a screwdriver.
Gym Use	Biceps curls, rows, throws, strikes.

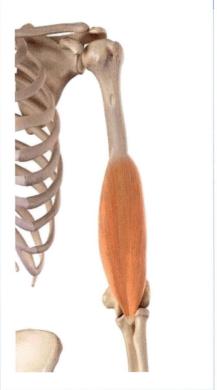

BRACHIORADIALIS

Origin	Humerus.
Insertion	Lower radius.
Action	Flexes the elbow, assists to pronate and supinate the forearm.
Antagonist	Triceps brachii.
Innervation	Radial nerve C5-C6.
Blood Supply	Radial, radial recurrent, and radial collateral artery.
Daily Use	Using a screwdriver, whisking an egg.
Gym Use	Reverse grip curls, throwing, grappling.

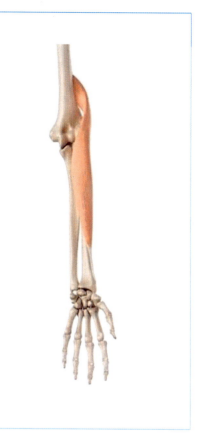

CORACOBRACHIALIS

Origin	Coracoid process of the scapula.
Insertion	Medial surface of the humerus.
Action	Flexes and adducts the shoulder.
Antagonist	Deltoid.
Innervation	Musculocutaneous nerve C5-C7.
Blood Supply	Brachial artery.
Daily Use	Raising your arms up to protect your face.
Gym Use	Dumbbell/cable fly.

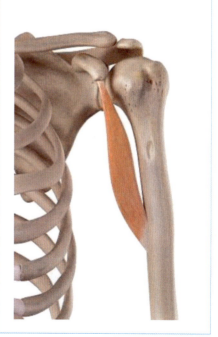

ROLLING THE BICEPS:

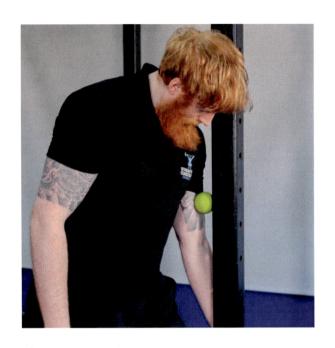

1. Hold a massage ball against a wall/post with one hand.
2. Hold your other arm straight down and allow it to relax completely.
3. Push the biceps of the straight arm into the massage ball. At this point, the ball should be supported by the biceps, and you can roll the surrounding muscle mass.
4. Slowly roll up and down the muscle for 30-60 seconds.
5. Complete 1-2 times on each side.

BARBELL ROLLING THE BICEPS:

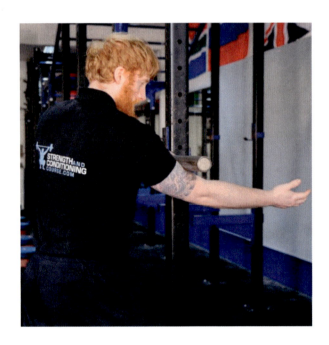

1. Set a barbell up on the rack at lower chest height
2. Hold the barbell down with one hand and raise your other arm up so that your biceps comes up to the sleeve of the barbell.
3. Slowly roll up and down the muscle for 30-60 seconds.
4. Complete 1-2 times on each side.

LYING BARBELL ROLLING THE BICEPS:

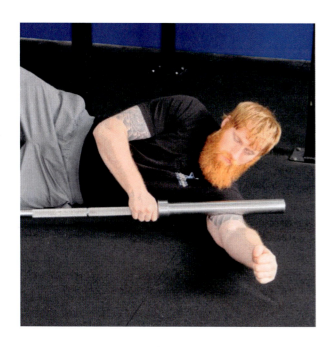

1. Place a barbell on the floor and lay on your side next to it.
2. Extend the arm you are lying on out to your front with your hand in a neutral position.
3. Allow your arm to relax completely.
4. Pick one end of the barbell up and place the sleeve onto your biceps.
5. Slowly roll up and down the muscle for 30-60 seconds.
6. Don't roll over the crease of your elbow.
7. You can also hold the barbell in place and slowly flex and extend your elbow 3-5 times to increase the release – this works well towards the top of your biceps close to where your deltoid inserts.
8. Complete 1-2 times on each side.

BICEPS WALL STETCH:

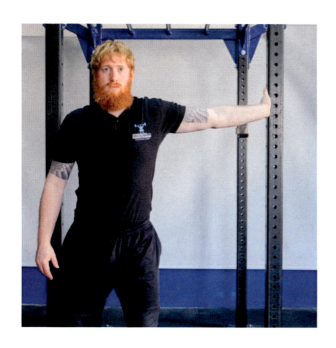

1. Stand side onto a wall/post, about an arms distance away.
2. With the arm closest to the wall, place your palm flat to the wall with your fingers facing rearwards.
3. Drive your palm/fingers into the wall/post and turn your biceps downwards without moving the position of your hand.
4. You can also rotate your body away from your arm to increase the stretch.
5. This stretch can feel incredibly intense as it is also targeting the median nerve.
6. Hold for 30-60 seconds, or 2 minutes if the musculature is very tense.
7. Complete 1-3 times on each side.

BAND BICEPS CURL:

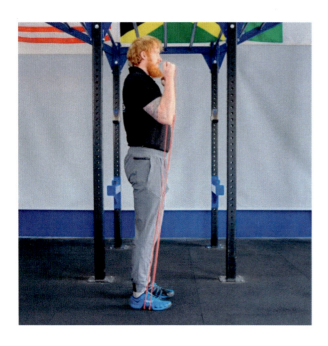

1. Use a low to medium-tension resistance band.
2. Grab the band in both hands and place one end of the band under the arches of both feet. Taking your feet wider will increase the band tension.
3. The band can also be placed around a solid structure to your front.
4. Hold the band at your side in a neutral grip (palms facing your legs).
5. Keep your upper body in good posture throughout the lift.
6. Contract your biceps, pulling the band upwards. As this happens, begin to supinate your forearms.
7. As you pass 90 degrees of elbow flexion, your elbows should come forward slightly to allow for a small amount of shoulder flexion.
8. Make a conscious effort to pull your little fingers in towards your chest. This maximizes the contraction at the top.
9. Lower under control, and don't swing rearwards as you come to the starting position.
10. Complete 2-3 sets of 10-20 reps.

FULL CURL:

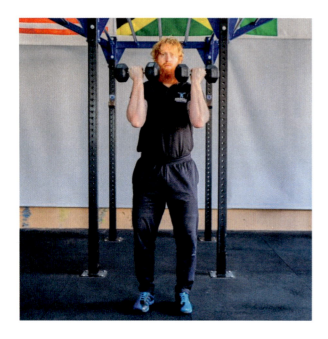

1. Stand up tall with good posture.
2. Hold the dumbbells at your side in a neutral grip – starting in a neutral grip allows you to supinate your forearms as you perform the curl, helping to increase biceps engagement.
3. Contract your biceps, bringing the dumbbells upwards, as this happens, begin to supinate your forearms.
4. As your elbows pass 90 degrees of flexion, bring your elbows forward slightly to increase the engagement of your biceps as you reach the top of the lift.
5. As you get to the top of the lift, supinate your palms as hard as you can to increase the engagement of the biceps – push your little fingers in towards your chest.
6. A shift grip (pictured) can be used to increase the work required to supinate your forearms.
7. Lower the dumbbells down under control to the starting position.
8. Don't swing the dumbbells rearwards.
9. Complete 2-3 sets of 10-15 reps.

HAMMER CURL:

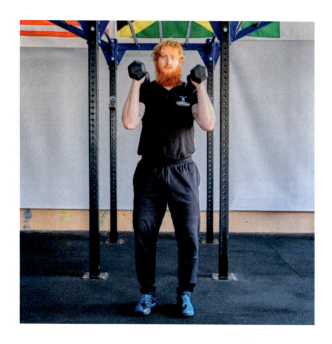

1. Stand up tall with good posture.
2. Hold the dumbbells at your side in a neutral grip.
3. Contract your biceps, bringing the dumbbells upwards.
4. Keep your hands in the neutral position.
5. As your elbows pass 90 degrees of flexion, bring your elbows forward slightly to increase the engagement of your biceps as you reach the top of the lift.
6. The top bell of the dumbbells should come up towards, or slightly above your shoulders. Squeeze your biceps hard at the top.
7. Lower the dumbbells down under control to the starting position.
8. Don't swing the dumbbells rearwards.
9. Complete 2-3 sets of 10 reps.

CROSSBODY HAMMER CURL:

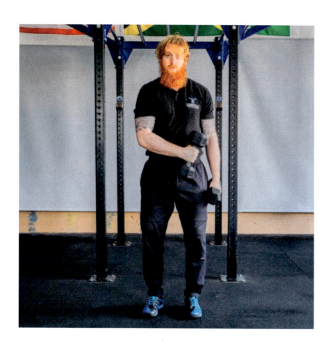

1. Stand up tall with good posture.
2. Hold the dumbbells at your side in a neutral grip.
3. Contract your biceps, bringing one dumbbell upwards and across your body.
4. Keep your hands in the neutral position (palms facing your body throughout).
5. Bring the dumbbell up towards your sternum (breastbone).
6. Lower the dumbbell down under control to the starting position and work the opposite side.
7. Don't use too much of a jerking action to throw the dumbbells up.
8. Complete 2-3 sets of 10 reps.

ZOTTMAN CURL:

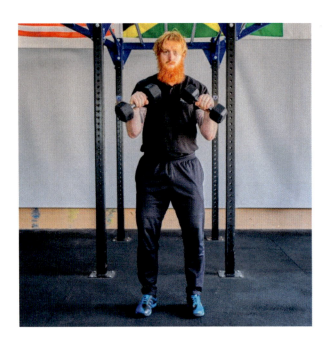

1. Stand up tall with good posture.
2. Hold the dumbbells at your side in a neutral grip.
3. Contract your biceps, bringing the dumbbells upwards, as this happens, supinate your forearms.
4. As your elbows pass 90 degrees of flexion, bring your elbows forward slightly to increase the engagement of your biceps as you reach the top of the lift.
5. As you get to the top of the lift, supinate your palms as hard as you can to increase the engagement of the biceps – push your little fingers in towards your chest.
6. At the top, rotate your wrists round so that your palms are facing forwards.
7. Lower the dumbbells down in a reverse curl position.
8. Don't swing the dumbbells rearwards.
9. Complete 2-3 sets of 10 reps.

THE TRICEPS

The triceps are a muscle group on the back of the arm and work to extend the elbow.

The long head of the triceps brachii also works to extend the shoulder as it attaches to the shoulder blade.

The triceps make up around two thirds of the upper arm and work incredibly hard during pressing exercises.

Many lifters will experience elbow pain. Therefore, it is key to manage training loads on the triceps and maintain good mobility in the muscle.

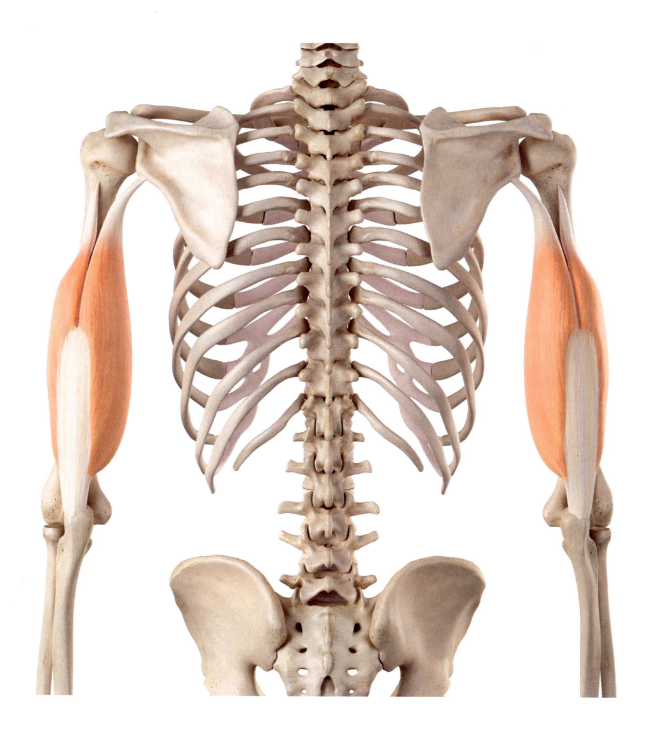

TRICEPS BRACHII	
Origin	Posterior upper humerus and scapula.
Insertion	Upper ulna.
Action	Extends the elbow and shoulder.
Antagonist	Biceps brachii.
Innervation	Radial nerve C6-C8.
Blood Supply	Deep brachial artery, posterior circumflex humeral artery (long head only).
Daily Use	Pushing a door closed, hammering a nail.
Gym Use	Push-ups, bench press, overhead press, triceps extensions, dips.

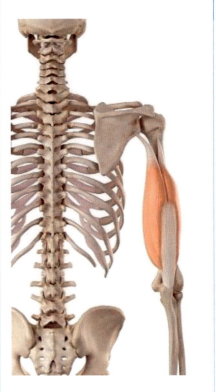

ROLLING THE TRICEPS:

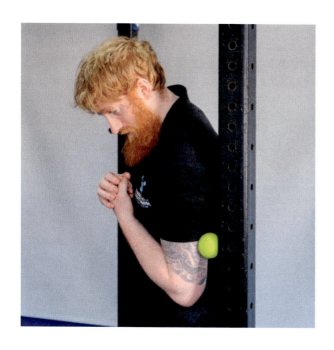

1. Hold a massage ball against a wall/post with one hand.
2. With your other arm, bend your elbow to relax your triceps.
3. Push the triceps of the bent arm into the massage ball. At this point, the ball should be supported by the triceps, and you can roll the surrounding muscle mass.
4. Slowly roll up and down the muscle for 30-60 seconds.
5. You can also flex and extend your elbow to increase the release.
6. Complete 1-2 times on each side.

BARBELL ROLLING THE TRICEPS:

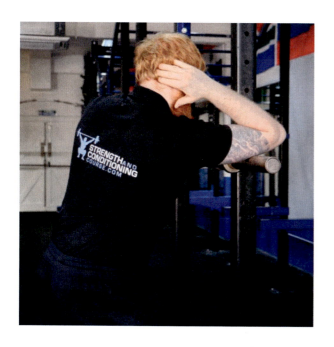

1. Set the barbell up on a rack at lower chest height.
2. Place the back of one arm onto the sleeve of the barbell while supporting yourself and the barbell with your other hand.
3. Slowly roll up and down the muscle for 30-60 seconds.
4. You can also flex and extend your elbow to increase the release.
5. Complete 1-2 times on each side.

STANDING TRICEPS STRETCH:

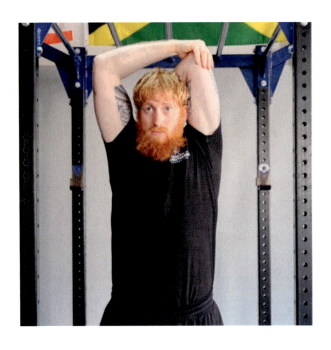

1. Stand upright with a hip-width stance.
2. Take your left arm overhead and reach down the center of your back.
3. Take your right arm and place it above your left elbow (on the triceps).
4. Pull on your left arm to pull it down and towards your right side
5. Hold for 30-60 seconds for a regular stretch or 2 minutes if the musculature is very tense.
6. Complete 1-3 times on each side.

WALL TRICEPS STRETCH:

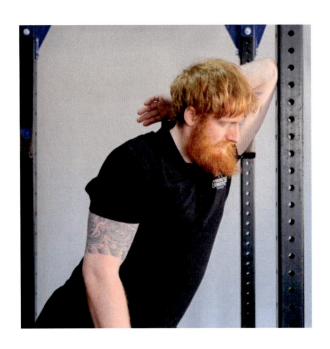

1. Bend your left elbow and bring your left hand over your right shoulder.
2. Place the back of your left arm on a wall or post and lean into it to apply a stretch.
3. Hold for 30-60 seconds for a regular stretch, or 2 minutes if the musculature is very tense.
4. Complete 1-3 times on each side.

TRICEPS EXTENSION:

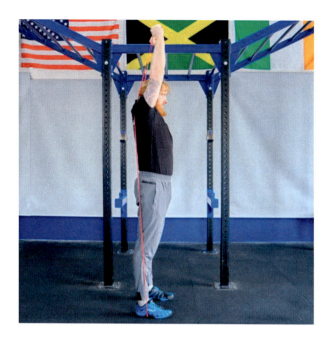

1. Use a low-tension resistance band (a weight plate or dumbbell can also be used).
2. Stand on the band and hold the other end behind your head.
3. Widening your stance will increase band tension.
4. Extend your arms overhead before slowly lowering your hands behind your head.
5. Complete 2-3 sets of 10-20 reps.

TRICEPS PUSHDOWN:

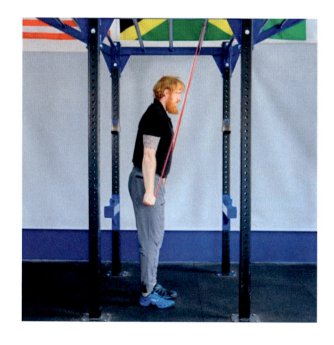

1. Use a low to medium-tension resistance band.
2. Attach the band to a solid structure overhead to perform the pushdown.
3. Hold the band at face height with a neutral grip. Your elbows should be slightly forward of your torso.
4. Keep your upper body in good posture throughout the lift.
5. Pull down on the band, keep your upper arms in line with your torso, and extend your elbows.
6. Don't jerk at your hips or lean over the band as you are pushing it down.
7. When using a neutral grip on the band, as you reach full extension of your elbows, turn your palms to face rearwards. This increases the contraction of your triceps.
8. Raise back up to the starting position under control.
9. Complete 2-3 sets of 10-20 reps.

THE FOREARMS

The forearm muscles can be split into two major groups, the flexors (on the palm side) and the extensors (on the dorsal side).

These muscles work to flex and extend the wrist and fingers and adduct and abduct the wrists.

The forearm muscles work incredibly hard during daily activities and within the gym. Therefore, if there is overuse, it can lead to elbow pain.

To prevent elbow pain, it is key to manage training loads and ensure both strength and mobility in the forearm muscles is maintained/developed.

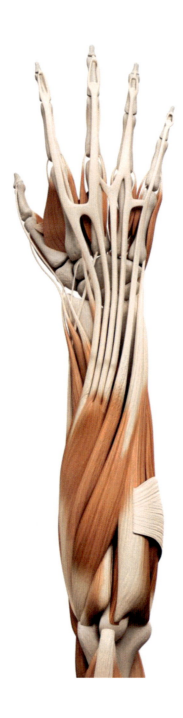

ROLLING THE FOREARMS:

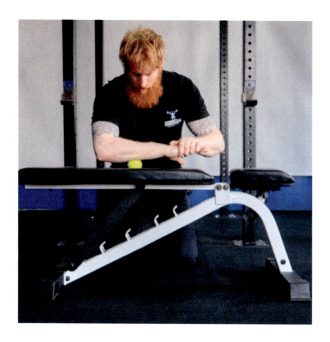

1. Place the massage ball (a foam roller can also be used) on a raised surface – bench or table.
2. Place your forearm onto the massage ball (flexors or extensors).
3. Slowly roll up and down the muscle for 30-60 seconds.
4. Complete 1-2 times on each side.

BARBELL ROLLING THE FOREARMS:

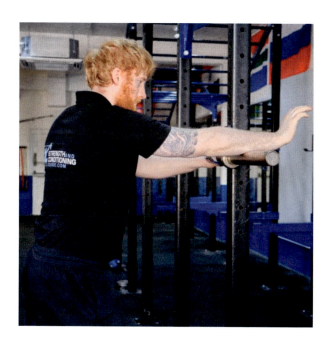

1. Set up a barbell up on a rack at around chest height – the barbell can be lowered to abdominal height if you find it easier to roll the tissues in this position.
2. Place your forearm on the sleeve of the barbell (on top for the flexors and underneath for the extensors).
3. Slowly roll up and down the muscle for 30-60 seconds.
4. Complete 1-2 times on each side.

SCRAPING THE FOREARMS:

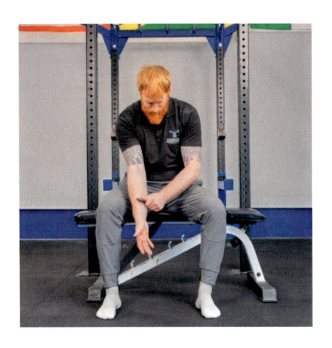

1. Hold the scraping tool in one hand and hold your other forearm to the front.
2. Scrape from your wrist to your elbow – we tend to massage towards the heart.
3. You can scrape both your flexors and extensors.
4. Scrape for 30-60 seconds on each side.

STANDING FLEXOR STRETCH:

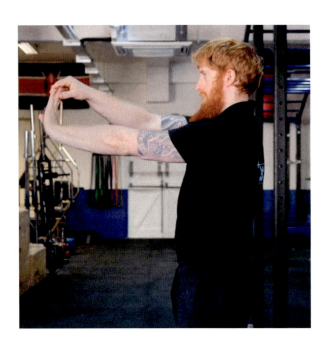

1. Stand upright in a hip-width stance.
2. Bring your right hand to the front, with your palm down, and point your fingers to the ceiling.
3. Grab your fingers with your left hand and pull back on them to apply a flexor stretch.
4. Hold for 30-60 seconds for a regular stretch, or 2 minutes if the musculature is very tense.
5. Complete 1-3 times on each side.

FLOOR FLEXOR STRETCH:

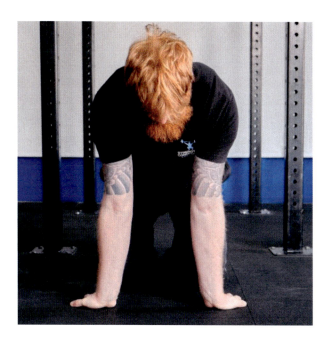

1. Kneel on the floor and place the palms of your hands on the floor with your fingers facing you.
2. Ensure the heel of your palms stays down and lean back to apply a stretch.
3. Hold for 30-60 seconds for a regular stretch, or 2 minutes if the musculature is very tense.
4. Complete 1-3 times.

STANDING EXTENSOR STRETCH:

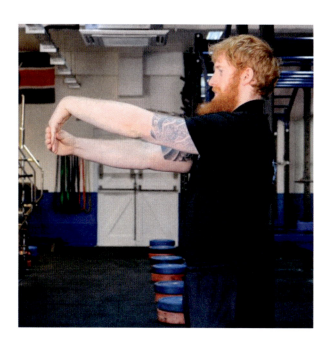

1. Stand upright in a hip-width stance.
2. Bring your right hand to the front, with your palm down, and point your fingers to the floor.
3. Grab your fingers with your left hand and pull back on them to apply an extensor stretch.
4. Hold for 30-60 seconds for a regular stretch, or 2 minutes if the musculature is very tense.
5. Complete 1-3 times on each side.

FLOOR EXTENSOR STRETCH:

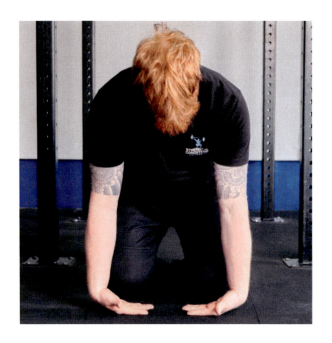

1. Kneel on the floor and place the back of your hands (dorsal side) on the floor with your fingers pointing towards each other.
2. Push down onto your hands to apply the stretch.
3. Hold for 30-60 seconds for a regular stretch, or 2 minutes if the musculature is very tense.
4. Complete 1-3 times.

BAND WRIST CURL:

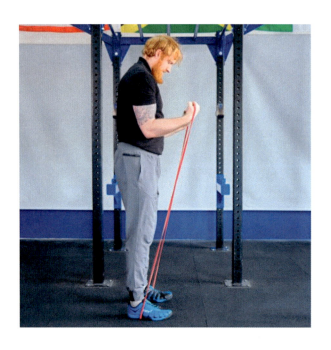

1. Stand on a low-medium tension band.
2. Hold the other end of the band in your hands and flex your elbows to 90 degrees to apply tension to the band.
3. If working the flexors, have your palms facing up or if working the extensors, have your palms facing the floor.
4. Curl your wrists upwards and ensure you are not compensating with the biceps – ensure your forearm muscles are doing the work.
5. Perform 2-3 sets of 10-20 reps on each side (or the side you are targeting).

DUMBBELL WRIST CURL:

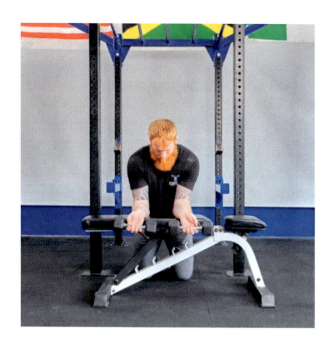

1. Hold a barbell or a small dumbbell in each hand.
2. Kneel and rest your forearms on a bench so your wrists are hanging over the other side of the bench – palms up to work the flexors or palms down to work the extensors.
3. Allow your hands to drop under control and the flex or extend your wrists to work the forearm muscles.
4. Complete 2-3 sets of 10-20 reps.

THE NECK

The neck is made up of 7 cervical vertebrae. The first vertebra is called the atlas, after the Greek god who supported the world on his shoulders. The second is called the axis. Together these make a pivot joint that allows the head to turn from side to side or rotate.

The neck is capable of flexion, which involves bringing your chin towards your chest. Lateral flexion, which involves bending your neck to the side and bringing your ear towards your shoulder. Extension, which involves bringing your head back to a straight position or looking towards the ceiling, and rotation, which, as mentioned previously, involves turning your head from side to side.

The muscles towards the front of the neck facilitate flexion, while the muscles towards the back facilitate extension. The other movements occur through unilateral contraction of the muscles to the front, rear and side of the neck.

Unilateral refers to one side. For example, raising one arm into the air is a unilateral movement, while raising two is a bilateral movement (opposite arm and leg = contralateral / same arm and leg = ipsilateral).

Most of our skeletal muscles come in pairs. Therefore, when one side works, it may produce the movement of one limb, a side bending, or rotational movement.

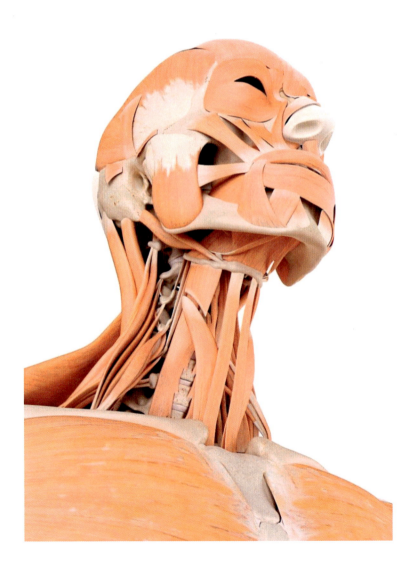

THE TRAPEZIUS

The trapezius (traps) is a large muscle on the upper back.

The traps are often split into three groups:

- Upper Traps.

- Middle (Mid) Traps.

- Lower Traps.

The upper traps mainly work to elevate the shoulder blades. The mid traps mainly work to retract the shoulder blades, and the lower traps mainly work to depress the shoulder blades.

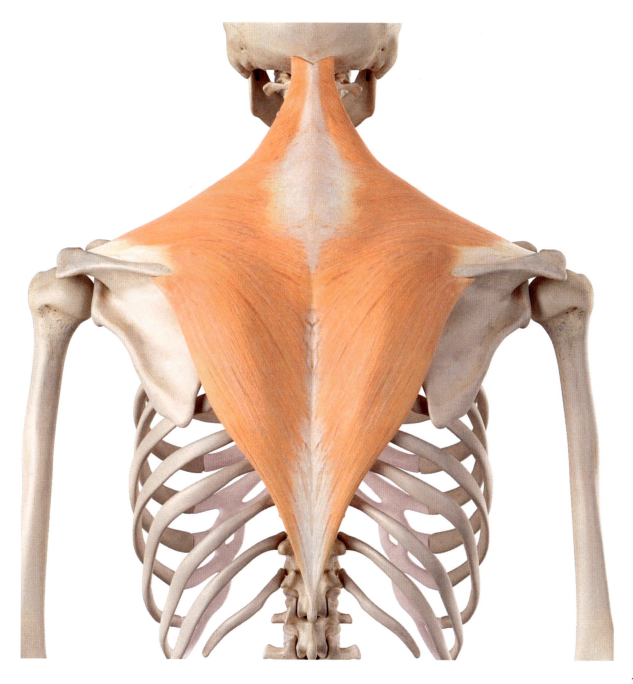

TRAPEZIUS	
Origin	Base of the skull and spinous processes of C7-T12.
Insertion	Lateral clavicle and upper surface of the scapula.
Action	Extends, adducts and internally rotates the shoulder.
Antagonist	Serratus anterior, latissimus dorsi and pectoralis major.
Innervation	Accessory nerve (motor), cervical spinal nerves C3-C4.
Blood Supply	Occipital, superficial or transverse cervical, and dorsal scapular arteries.
Daily Use	Shrugging your shoulders, picking up a heavy object.
Gym Use	Shrugs, upright rows, deadlifts.

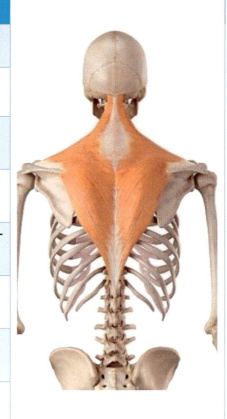

ROLLING THE TRAPEZIUS:

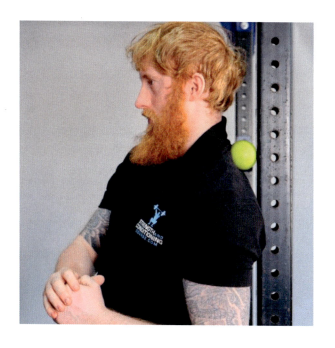

1. Standing: Place the massage ball on a wall/post, and while holding it with one hand, push your back into it to support the ball (this can be a little awkward).
2. Roll the ball into position.
3. Lying: Place the massage ball on the floor.
4. Lie onto the massage ball so that it is pushed into your lower-mid trap.
5. Knead the tissues for around 30-60 seconds.
6. Complete 1-2 times on each side.

UPPER TRAPEZIUS RELEASE:

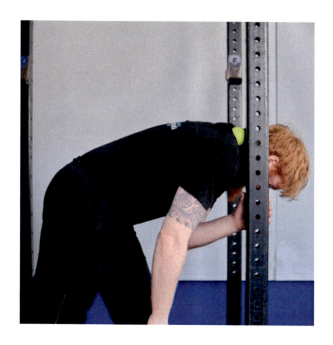

1. Place a massage ball against a post, bend over and push your upper trap into the ball.
2. To aid in the release, you can move the arm on the side that is being released. For example, flex, extend, abduct, adduct, and circumduct your shoulder.
3. Knead the tissues for around 30-60 seconds.
4. Complete 1-2 times on each side.

BARBELL TRAPEZIUS RELEASE:

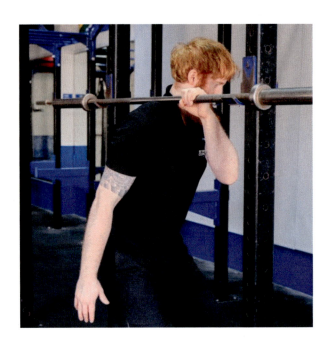

1. Set a barbell up on a rack at mid-upper chest height.
2. This drill is best done with 15kg+ plates on either side to weight the barbell down.
3. Stand side onto the barbell, bend underneath and push your trapezius up into the barbell.
4. Hold this position for 30-60 seconds and gently move your neck through various actions (lateral flexion and extension and rotation).
5. During this time, you can also move the arm on the side you are releasing through various actions.
6. Complete 1-2 times on each side.

STANDING TRAPEZIUS STRETCH:

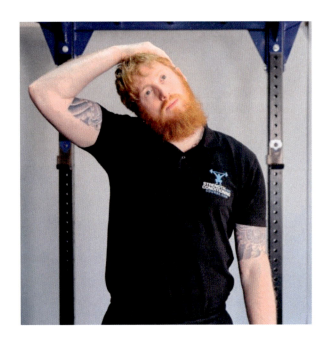

1. Stand up and slowly bring your ear towards your right shoulder.
2. Grab above your left ear with your right hand and hold a gentle stretch for 20-30 seconds
3. To increase the stretch, lean your body slightly towards the left to depress your shoulder further (push down with your left hand – as if putting it in your pocket).
4. Complete 1-3 times on each side.

SEATED TRAPEZIUS STRETCH:

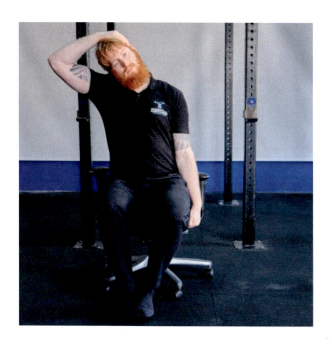

1. Sit with your chest up and hold onto the chair seat with your left hand.
2. Slowly bring your ear towards your right shoulder.
3. Grab above your left ear with your right hand and hold a gentle stretch for 20-30 seconds
4. To increase the stretch, lean your body slightly towards the right to depress your shoulder further.
5. Complete 1-3 times on each side.

SHRUGS:

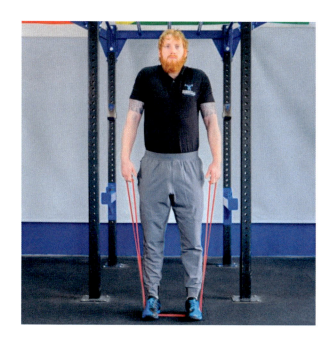

1. Stand upright in good posture.
2. Hold each end of a low to medium-tension resistance band in your hands and stand in the middle of it.
3. Brace your core.
4. Without bending your elbows shrug your shoulders upwards as high as you can. Don't work in a circular motion, only up and down.
5. Ensure your shoulders are driving upwards and you are not driving your head and back downwards.
6. It often works better to inhale during the upwards phase of the lift rather than during the downward phase (this is the opposite to most strength exercises) – it feels more natural to have your ribcage expanding as you shrug your shoulders.
7. Hold the top position for a second or two before slowly lowering the shoulders back down to the starting position and complete successive reps.
8. Complete 2-3 sets of 10-20 reps.

UPRIGHT ROWS:

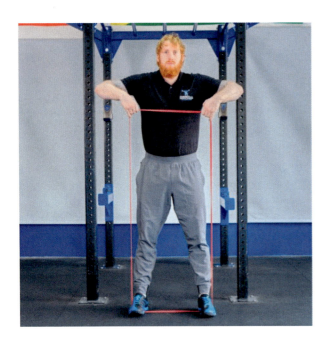

1. Stand upright in good posture.
2. Stand on the inside of a low to medium-tension band and hold the top end with a narrow shoulder-width grip – a wider grip is less stressful on the shoulders.
3. Brace your core.
4. Pull upwards and outwards with your elbows to pull the band up while keeping the band as close to the body as possible – keep your wrists lower than your elbows (don't turn them over).
5. Hold the top position for a second or two before slowly lowering the shoulders back down to the starting position and complete successive reps.
6. Complete 2-3 sets of 10-20 reps.

DEEP NECK EXTENSORS

The neck extensors include the upper trapezius, but also deeper muscles such as the splenius capitis and splenius cervicis.

Muscles on the back of the neck can become tense causing discomfort and even headaches. Therefore, the right release techniques and stretches can be hugely beneficial.

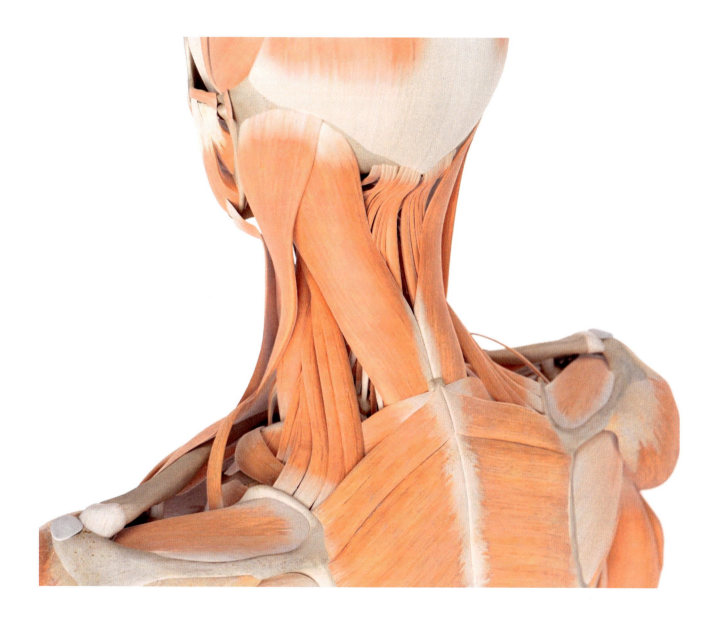

ROLLING THE DEEP NECK EXTENSORS:

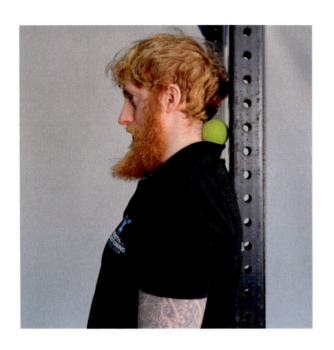

1. Standing: Place the massage ball or peanut ball on a wall/post, and while holding it with one hand, push your neck into it to support the ball (this can be a little awkward).
2. Lying: Place the massage ball on the floor.
3. Lie onto the massage ball so that it is pushed into the back of your neck.
4. Knead the tissues for 30-60 seconds.
5. Complete 1-2 times.

DEEP NECK EXTENSOR STRETCH:

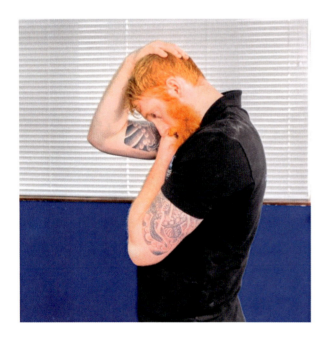

1. Sit with your chest up and look straight ahead.
2. Gently push your chin back with your hand (so that you have a double chin)
3. While holding your chin back with one hand, use your other hand to reach over the top of your head.
4. Stabilize your chin as you gently pull the top of your head forward and hold a gentle stretch for 20-30 seconds.
5. Complete 1-3 times.

HAND RESISTED NECK ISO HOLDS:

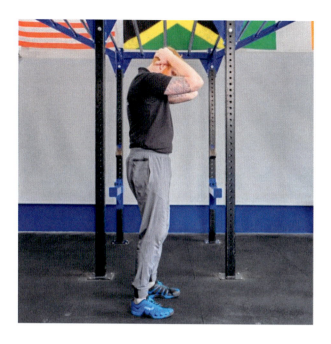

1. Place one or both hands at any position on your head (forehead, back of head, side of head).
2. Push your head back into your hand(s) for 5-15 seconds.
3. Perform 2-3 sets of 5-15 seconds holds.

BAND NECK ISO HOLDS:

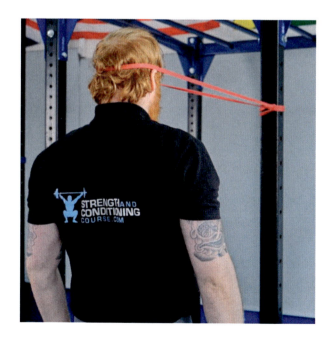

1. Use a low-tension resistance band. The tension can be varied by standing closer or further away from the band attachment point.
2. Attach the band to a solid structure at head height.
3. Wrap a small towel around the part of the band which goes around your head as the rubber band can pull on your hair.
4. Place the band around your head (above your ears) and step away from the attachment point to add tension to the band.
5. You can stand facing the band attachment point, with your back to it, with your right or left side facing it, or at an oblique angle from the band attachment point to work the different areas of the neck.
6. Ensure that your feet, hips, shoulders, and head are forward facing. Don't counter the band tension by turning away from the attachment point.
7. Engage your core, create tension in your upper back and neck and hold the position for 30-40 seconds.

THE LEVATOR SCAPULA

The levator scapula as the name suggests work to elevate the scapula. It also works to laterally flex and extend the neck.

Forward head posture puts increased tension on the levator scapula muscle. Therefore, release techniques and stretches can be useful for this muscle.

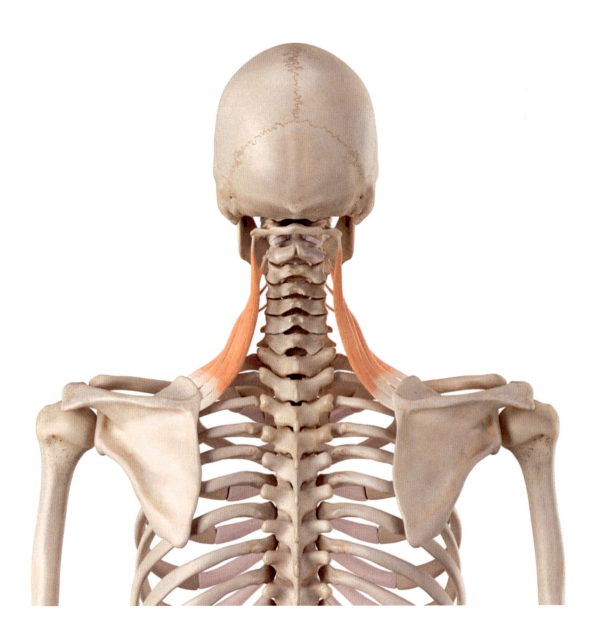

LEVATOR SCAPULA	
Origin	Transverse processes of C1-C4.
Insertion	Superior angle of the scapula.
Action	Elevates the shoulder girdle, laterally flexes and extends the neck.
Antagonist	Serratus anterior and middle trapezius.
Innervation	Cervical nerve C3-C4, and dorsal scapular nerve C5.
Blood Supply	Transverse cervical and ascending cervical arteries.
Daily Use	Looking over your shoulder, carrying a bag.
Gym Use	Shrugs, upright rows, deadlifts.

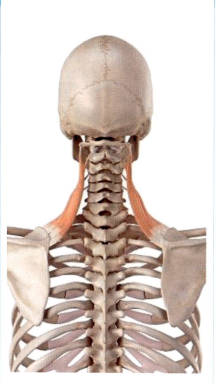

ROLLING THE LEVATOR SCAPULA:

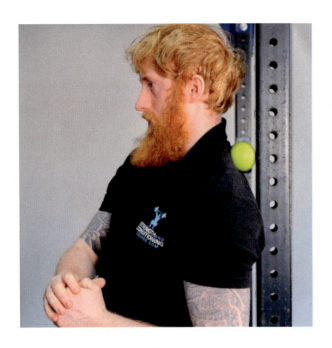

1. Standing: Place the massage ball on a wall/post, and while holding it with one hand, push your upper back-neck into it to support the ball (this can be a little awkward).
2. Roll the ball into position.
3. Lying: Place the massage ball on the floor.
4. Lie onto the massage ball so that it is pushed into your upper back-neck.
5. Knead the tissues for around 30-60 seconds.
6. Complete 1-2 times on each side.

LEAVTOR SCAPULA STRETCH:

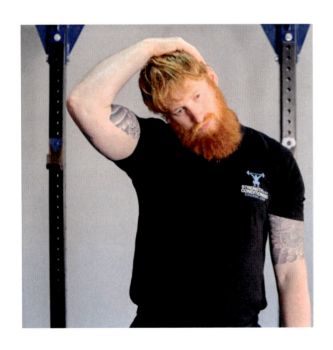

1. Stand up with a hip-width stance – this can also be done in a chair like the seated trap stretch.
2. Slowly look towards your right pants pocket.
3. Hold the back, left side of your head with your right hand, and hold a gentle stretch for 20-30 seconds.
4. Complete 1-3 times on each side.

SCALENES AND STERNOCLEIDOMASTOID (SCM)

The scalenes and sternocleidomastoid (SCM) are muscles on the side and front of the neck. They work to flex, laterally flex, and extend the neck.

Forward head posture puts increased tension on these muscles. Therefore, release techniques and stretches can be useful for these muscles.

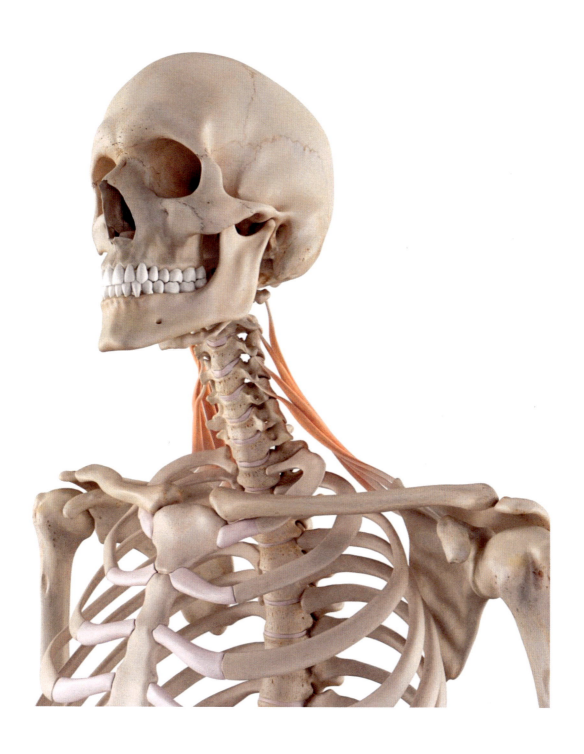

SCALENES	
Origin	Anterior: Transverse processes of vertebrae C3-C6 / Middle: C2-C7 / Posterior: C5-C7.
Insertion	Anterior and middle: Rib 1 / Posterior: Rib 2.
Action	Flexion and lateral flexion of the neck and elevation of rib 1 and 2.
Antagonist	Semispinalis capitis and cervicis, splenius capitis and cervicis, spinalis cervicis.
Innervation	Anterior rami of spinal nerves.
Blood Supply	Ascending cervical branch of the inferior thyroid artery.
Daily Use	Bending your head to one side.
Gym Use	Neck curls and stabilization.

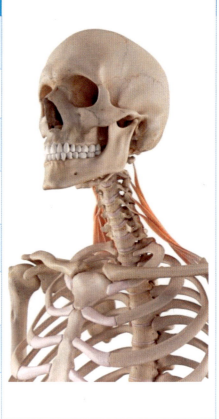

STERNOCLEIDOMASTOID	
Origin	Sternal head: The manubrium sterni / Clavicular head: Superior surface of the clavicle.
Insertion	Mastoid process of the temporal bone, superior nuchal line.
Action	Unilaterally: Cervical rotation, cervical flexion / Bilaterally: cervical flexion, elevation of sternum.
Antagonist	Longus capitis, rectus capitis anticus.
Innervation	Accessory nerve, branches of cervical plexus (C2-C3).
Blood Supply	Occipital artery and the superior thyroid artery.
Daily Use	Turning your head.
Gym Use	Neck curls and stabilization.

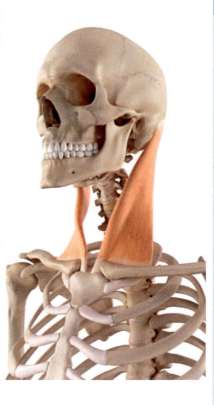

SCALENE AND STRENOCLEIDOMASTOID STRETCH:

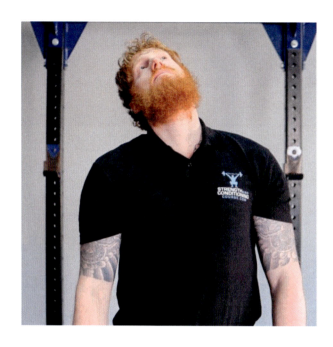

1. Sit or stand with your chest up.
2. Rotate your head slightly toward your left.
3. Side bend your head to the right and look upwards as you do so.
4. Hold a gentle stretch for 20-30 seconds.
5. Repeat on the opposite side.
6. Complete 1-3 times on each side.

BAND NECK ISO HOLDS:

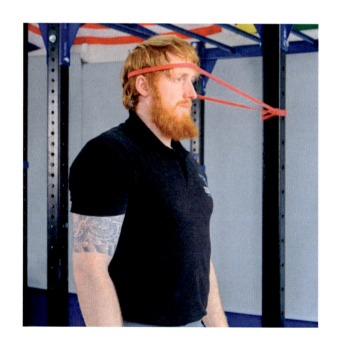

1. Use a low-tension resistance band. The tension can be varied by standing closer or further away from the band attachment point.
2. Attach the band to a solid structure at head height.
3. Wrap a small towel around the part of the band which goes around your head as the rubber band can pull on your hair.
4. Place the band around your head (above your ears) and step away from the attachment point to add tension to the band.
5. You can stand facing the band attachment point, with your back to it, with your right or left side facing it, or at an oblique angle from the band attachment point to work the different areas of the neck.
6. Ensure that your feet, hips, shoulders and head are forward facing. Don't counter the band tension by turning away from the attachment point.
7. Engage your core, create tension in your upper back and neck and hold the position for 30-40 seconds.

LOWER-BODY COMPOUND MOVEMENTS

Lower body compound movement are split into four major categories:

- **Hinge:** Exercises that emphasize hip flexion and extension.

- **Squat:** Exercises where the hips and knees bend to lower the body into a squat.

- **Lunge:** Single-leg exercises.

- **Gait:** Walking, running and loaded carries.

Especially when worked with free weights (barbells, dumbbells, and kettlebells), most of the exercises will work the entire body to some extent.

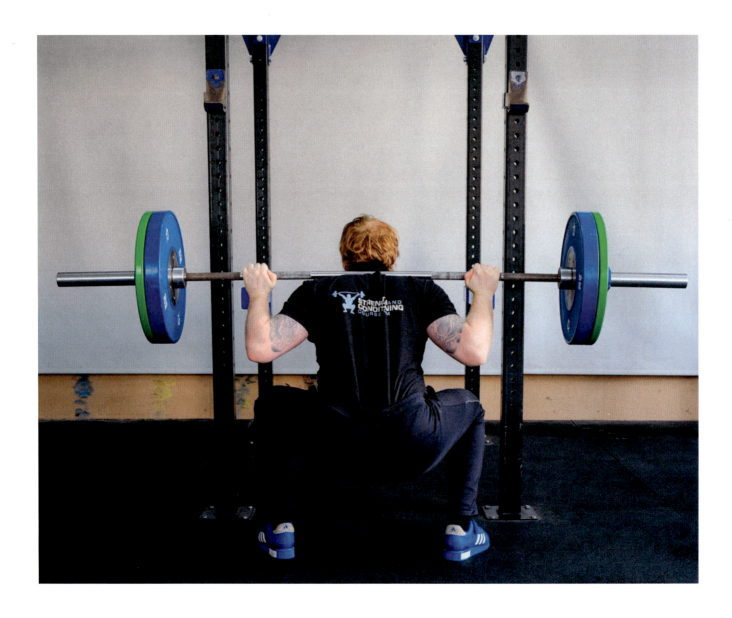

THE HINGE

The hinge involves bending at the hips to bring your torso forward while maintaining a neutral spine. Of course, we can bend or twist our spine as we hinge. However, when lifting heavy loads, we aim to align ourselves into the optimal posture, minimizing the risk of injury and maximizing performance.

The hip hinge can be quite awkward, and individuals will often perform the movement with excessive flexion of the spine or/and too much knee bend.

Here are the basic teaching points I begin with:

1. Stand with soft knees (slightly bent) and good upper body posture, ensuring your chest is proud (pushed out) and remains so throughout the movement.

2. Start by driving your glutes backward.

3. Maintain the soft knee position and keep driving your glutes back. This will cause your hips to hinge, bringing your torso forward.

4. Keep going until you feel your hamstrings reach the extent of their range of motion and ensure you maintain a neutral spine – if you don't feel the stretch in your hamstrings, you are not pushing your hips back enough.

5. With straight legs (soft knees) and maintaining a neutral spine, this will usually bring your torso to parallel or just above parallel to the floor.

Methods of correcting faults:

- Have the client exaggerate a proud chest position for 5-10 seconds (push the chest out hard). This allows them to feel the erector spinae muscles' engagement, which keeps the spine in extension.

- Stand the client about a foot's distance in front of a wall while maintaining a proud chest, cue them to touch the wall with their glutes. This drill is perfect for teaching clients to shift their hips/glutes backward to maximize the hamstrings and glutes' engagement and can be progressed by standing further away from the wall.

- Use a dowel placed on the client's back. There should be 3 points of contact, the back of the head, between the shoulder blades, and on the sacrum. If these 3 points of contact are lost during the hinge, the client is rounding their spine.

- Place a resistance band around the client's hips and while standing behind them, pull on the band to encourage the hips to move backward as the torso tilts. This can also be done with a band attached to a solid structure, stepping away from the attachment point to create band tension that will pull the client's hips back. The band tension also promotes a stronger hip extension.

- Have the client hold a kettlebell behind their back. This can help to ensure they maintain a proud chest.

One of the most common faults is being too far away from the weight when working with weights. Therefore, a lifter should aim to stand right over or just behind the weight.

One of the most common faults we see when progressing to barbell deadlifts is not keeping the barbell close enough. This is often just poor technique in general, and the right cues will usually sort the issue, such as "pull the bar in" or "hide your armpits." However, it is also down to a lack of latissimus dorsi engagement as a whole, which can be worked on with specific drills and exercises.

The lats are a considerable muscle mass and work to extend the shoulders. Therefore, as the hips are extending into the barbell, the lats should be extending the shoulders to keep the barbell close, pulling it into the hips.

We can increase lat engagement with:

- Band lat pulls downs.

- Band straight arm lat pulldowns.

We can also use a resistance band during deadlifts to reinforce the optimal positioning. For this, we attach a band to a post and then around the centre of a barbell set up with plates. From there, we perform deadlifts while the band is trying to pull the barbell away from us – this is a Reactive Neuromuscular Technique (RNT).

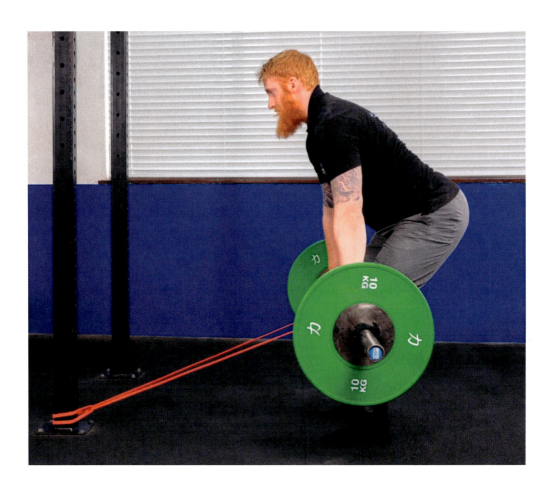

KB/DB DEADLIFT

To progress the bodyweight hinge, we add a little bit of weight and the easiest way to do this is with a kettlebell (KB) or dumbbell (DB) on the floor.

Suppose an individual is struggling to maintain a straight back. In that case, it works well to exaggerate the proud chest position and perform the deadlift like a sumo squat (it is still technically a deadlift if the weight is going dead on the floor).

I will usually progress this drill by having the client begin by taking a wide stance directly over the KB or DB and tell them to squat down while keeping the chest proud and the back as upright as possible. This setup is easy to master and will place more load on the quads and adductors while a stiff back position is ingrained. From there, the client progressively (set by set) brings their feet closer together and emphasizes the hip hinge rather than the knee bend – this is by far the most effective method I have found to in-still a rigid torso while hinging at the hips.

The exercise can also be performed from a deficit by standing on two weight plates, turning the exercise into a sumo deficit squat – a deficit is a great way to increase the range of motion of hinge and squat exercises with a DB or KB held below the hips.

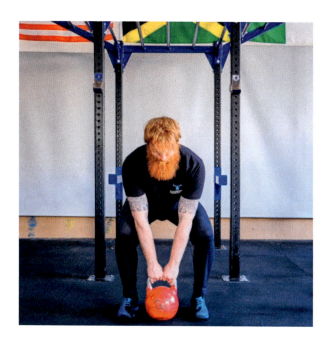

1. Place a kettlebell or dumbbell (KB/DB) on the floor.
2. Stand over the KB/DB in a hip-width to shoulder-width stance or a much wider sumo stance – a sumo stance works the quads and adductors harder, white a narrow stance works the posterior chain harder.
3. Bend at the hips and knees – ensure you sit back with your glutes.
4. While keeping your arms straight, grab the handle (horn) of the KB or the top bell of the DB.
5. Drive your feet into the floor and stand up while keeping your arms straight.
6. Complete 2-3 sets of 10-15 reps.

ROMANIAN DEADLIFT

The Romanian deadlift came about when weightlifters in a gym in San Francisco saw the Romanian lifter Nicu Vlad performing the lift. They asked him what the lift was called, and he replied, "back strengthening exercise," so they named it the Romanian Deadlift or RDL for short.

During a true RDL, the hips are not fully locked out at the top, which keeps the tension on the muscles and maximizes the need for a strong back. However, it is OK to lockout at the top to maximize glute engagement. Doing so in an explosive fashion is often referred to as a "Dimel deadlift," an exercise named after the late Matt Dimel, a renowned Powerlifter from Westside Barbell, an infamous gym in Columbus, Ohio.

As mentioned, weightlifters don't fully lockout during the RDL to keep tension on the back muscles. They also tend to develop explosive hip extension with snatch and clean pull variations.

The RDL is my lift of choice when progressing individuals from a bodyweight hinge and KB/DB deadlift to working with the barbell, and it acts as the ideal prerequisite to the deadlift.

To perform the RDL, we hold the barbell at the top of a deadlift, hinge at our hips, and allow the barbell to tack smoothly down our thighs. Once the barbell passes the kneecaps, we bend the knees slightly to bring the barbell 3-4 inches below the knees before reversing the movement and returning to the starting position.

The slight bend in the knees slacks the hamstrings and places emphasis on the back and glutes.

When performing the RDL, the lifter must initiate the movement by pushing their glutes back and allowing their shoulders to come forward of the barbell, enabling the barbell to track smoothly down the thighs. However, if the shoulders are kept behind the barbell, the barbell will get stuck on the thighs.

During an RDL, the lifter should turn their elbows into the plates, grip the floor with their feet (think heel, big toe, and the little toe), and push their knees out slightly to maximize the tension in the legs.

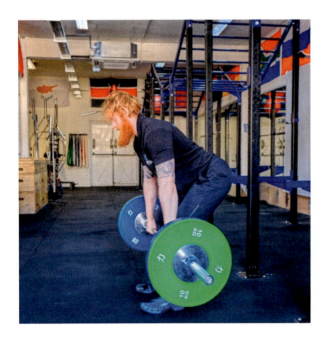

1. Start with the barbell at your hips with a pronated (overhand) grip.
2. Initiate the movement by driving your glutes back and bending your knees slightly. Allow your shoulders to come over the barbell while it maintains contact with your legs.
3. Keep driving your glutes back to facilitate the hinge and allow the barbell to track down your quads.
4. Once the barbell passes your kneecaps, bend your knees slightly to bring the barbell to about a palm's distance below your knees.
5. Engage your posterior chain and bring the barbell back up your legs, following the same path it went down. Maintain a vertical bar path throughout.
6. If locking out at the top, squeeze your glutes hard at the top before proceeding with successive reps.
7. Complete 3-5 sets of 5-10 reps.

ROTATIONAL ROMANIAN DEADLIFT (RRDL)

The rotational RDL (RRDL) is an exercise I use with all my lifters to build resilience in the lower back and keep any lower back stiffness out the way, specifically associated with the sacroiliac joints (SIJ), which are made up between the sacrum and ilium.

When lifters perform lots of heavy squats and deadlifts, primarily working through the sagittal plane, they can become stiff through the transverse plane, which is often felt around the lower back and SIJs.

Performing a hinge exercise with a slight rotation is a great way to apply torsion onto the joints and release any unwanted tension.

The RRDL can be practiced from blocks, which is essentially a rotational deadlift. This is an excellent way to tailor the range and overall stress on the lower back, allowing you to build back strength with minimal negative stress on the structures.

Once sufficient back strength is developed to accommodate the stress, you can progress onto the full RRDL, where the load is kept off the floor or blocks for the entire set.

To perform the RRDL, stand in a hip-width stance and hold a dumbbell or kettlebell in both hands. From there, hinge your hips and rotate the weight to one side, bringing the weight towards the outer side of the heel of one leg. As this happens, the other leg's knee bends slightly to allow for a greater range of rotation.

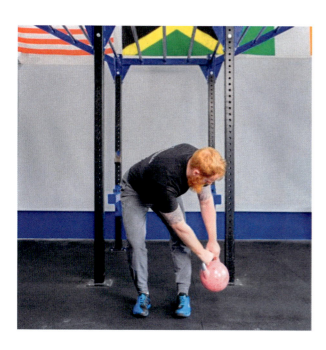

1. Pick a kettlebell or dumbbell up with both hands and stand in a narrow hip-width stance – with straight arms, the weight should hang just below your groin.
2. Hip hinge and rotate the weight to the outer side of your right foot (keep the weight off the floor).
3. As you hinge and take the weight towards the outer side of your right foot, bend your left knee slightly to increase the range of motion.
4. Engage your posterior chain muscles to raise back up to the starting position.
5. Complete 2-3 sets of 5-10 reps to each side.

THE DEADLIFT

The deadlift is the king of the hinge and pull movements, and is fundamental to the development of strong, powerful hips.

Please note that lifting a heavy weight off the floor can stress your spine in a way that can cause injury. It is essential that you perform this exercise with good form.

It should be noted, however, that injuries are not just a matter of technique or poor form. Regardless of whether you lift correctly or not, if your soft tissues haven't got the strength to handle the load (even with perfect form), injuries such as straining your lower back muscles can occur.

When it comes to the deadlift, many people are hell-bent on going as heavy as they can on every session, even if it's the first time they have lifted a barbell off the floor. However, to make real physical progression, you need to develop every link within the kinetic chain that is your body and *progressive programming* (gradually becoming harder) will allow all your structures to adapt, remembering that some structures (particularly smaller muscles involved in joint stabilisation) may not develop as quickly as others.

The lower back is one of the most important links within the kinetic chain. Without strength in this area, we not only compromise performance, but also risk serious, life-changing injury.

Do not underestimate the importance of the lower back – it truly is an integral part of your ability to maintain posture and maximise performance.

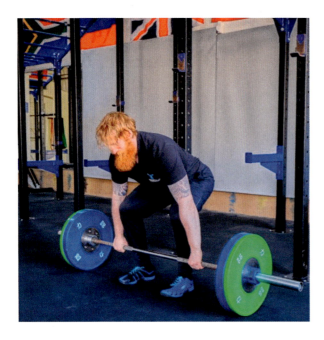

1. Stand with your midfoot under the barbell.
2. Hinge at your hips, bend your knees and grab the barbell.
3. Take a pronated or alternated grip. Use a pronated grip as much as possible.
4. Sit back with your glutes and drive your chest up. This will bring your shins forward.
5. Take a big gulp of air, brace your core, and use the Valsalva manoeuvre. As you do this, pull on the barbell to take away the slack and create total body tension.
6. Drive your heels into the floor and pull the barbell upwards and rearwards off the floor.
7. Once the barbell passes your knees, drive your hips into it and push your chest up. Your shoulders will fall naturally behind the barbell.
8. At the top, reverse the movement back down – keep the barbell on your legs.
9. At the bottom, exhale and get ready for the next rep.
10. Complete 3-5 sets of 1-5 reps.

THE SQUAT

Squats are the foundation of strength development and should be incorporated in some way into everyone's training regime. Whether it be a young child, teenager, 40-year-old couch potato, 20-year-old elite level athlete, or retired 75-year-old, all will benefit from moving and building strength in the legs.

A child will build good movement, balance, and coordination from performing a bodyweight squat. An older adult will benefit from performing box squats to build the strength to get up out of a chair. An athlete will dramatically increase their ability to produce maximal force while performing heavy front squats.

There is a lot of debate regarding the correct depth for a squat. Some argue it necessary to bend their hips, knees, and ankles fully (go ass to grass), which is essential for Olympic weightlifters. While others suggest squatting to a parallel (thighs in relation to the floor) or just below parallel to be ideal – in Powerlifting, an athlete must go just below parallel (break parallel) for the squat to count.

Joint anatomy and limb lengths play a crucial role in how people squat, and ultimately it comes down to the individual and their goals.

To effectively build strength in a muscle or muscle group, we want to work a muscle through its full range of motion as mechanically this elicits the greatest stress. However, we also want to maximize the force, speed, and power we can produce, which is not always possible from a depth where the joints are fully bent.

There are three points to consider when deciding how to perform a movement:

- Maximize the weight that can be lifted, i.e., maximize performance.

- Maximize the work required by the muscles (positive stress).

- Minimize the negative stress placed on the supporting structures.

Most individuals will look for a balance between maximizing the loads that can be lifted while working through a decent range of motion. Therefore, a squat that breaks parallel (top of kneecaps higher than the hips' crease) can be considered the "conventional squat depth." However, there is no reason why a lifter can't spend one session working a squat through a full range (ass to grass) and another working with heavier loads to a parallel position or even a partial range squat above parallel.

Optimal depth all comes down to finding the optimal balance to achieve the best results for your body and chosen sport, and this varies from person to person because their strengths, weaknesses, and needs differ.

BODYWEIGHT SQUAT

The bodyweight squat is something everyone should be able to perform. However, it is surprising how many people struggle with such a fundamental movement pattern.

The bodyweight squat is usually the first movement I have an individual perform because it acts as a great movement screening.

When teaching the bodyweight squat, I often don't overload the individual with information. I simply instruct them to:

- Take a shoulder-width stance.

- Sit back with your glutes (bum) and bend your knees.

- Bring your hands to your front and go to a depth that feels right.

From there, I progress specifically to any issues I have just picked up, and if they performed a perfect squat, I tell them why and progress it.

Remember, the first step to correcting a fault is the conscious engagement of the correct form.

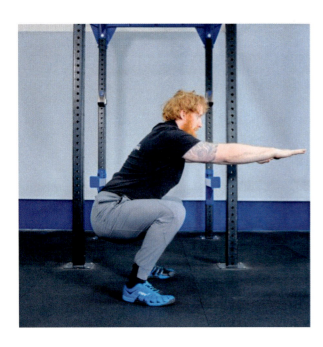

1. Take a shoulder-width stance – the stance someone chooses comes down to joint structures, limb lengths, and personal preference.
2. Toes are either pointing forwards or angled out slightly (usually at around 20-30 degrees).
3. Initiate the squat by bending at the hips (sit back with the glutes) and bend the knees almost simultaneously.
4. Keep the knees in line with the toes.
5. Keeping the trunk muscles engaged will reduce lumbar flexion at the bottom (butt wink).
6. A great cue is to imagine your torso dropping between your legs.
7. A common cue is to drive through the heels as you come up. This maximizes the posterior chain's engagement (hamstrings, glutes, etc) and is great if someone tends to come onto their toes. However, we should also ensure we have good contact with our big and little toes (Think: heel, big toe, little toe).
8. Complete 2-3 sets of 10-15 reps.

LACK OF DEPTH AND EXCESSIVE FORWARD LEAN

If someone is struggling with depth, we can do a few things to improve this instantly. However, not all changes happen overnight, and therefore, just because someone isn't breaking any records when it comes to squat depth, it doesn't mean all squats need to be cancelled in exchange for a rigid mobility regime.

Note: One of the easiest ways to increase depth is to raise the heel on a 1-2.5cm block.

When we squat, our centre of mass is shifted backward (sitting back with the hips). Therefore, people will often compensate for this by tilting their torso forward, which acts as a counterbalance (therefore putting your hands to the front can help). Excessive forward lean is a common fault and can be exacerbated by tight calves, hamstrings, hip flexors, and weak erector spinae muscles. However, although poor mobility is often an issue, people will jump to the conclusion that a lack of depth is down to poor flexibility when, it is merely a technique and stability issue.

The best way to see if this is the case is to use a small weight held to the front as a counterbalance, i.e., a goblet squat. The goblet squat can take someone from terrible form to great form in a couple of sets – it is incredible how a little bit of load can make a movement feel more stable and less flimsy.

Note: Unfortunately, long femurs (thigh bones) are not optimal levers for squatting and can exacerbate the torso's forward lean – skeletal structure is not something we are going to change.

The steps to achieving greater depth:

Initial fixes:

- Pause and increase depth – squat down and hold the position and then make a conscious effort to go a little further (you will be amazed at how well this works).

- The goblet squat – a counterbalance is key!

- Roll the soles of the feet and calves – this causes a short-term neurological effect that releases the tissues up the back of the leg and allows for greater dorsiflexion.

Long-term mobility:

- Couch Stretch.

- Hamstring Stretches.

- Heel Drop Calf Stretch.

- Deep Squat Stretch.

GOBLET SQUAT

The goblet squat is an excellent variation that will help you to develop your squat mechanics.

This exercise was invented by strength coach Dan John and was named after the way the weight is held high at the chest as if holding a large goblet.

When novices perform bodyweight squats with little depth and excessive forward tilt of their torso, coaches often try to rectify any perceived mobility issues. However, stability, not mobility, is often the underlying problem, as the person compensates for their centre of mass shifting rearwards.

A coach should give the novice a weight to hold, and the goblet position makes a perfect counterbalance to the weight of the body moving backward. The weight removes many stability issues and allows for greater depth to be achieved as their torso remains more upright. The goblet squat can progress someone with a terrible bodyweight squat to squatting well within one set.

For a goblet squat, a kettlebell is usually used, but dumbbells (cup the top bell of the dumbbell in your hands) or weight plates also work well.

When performing goblet squats, you should keep your elbows tucked in so that your elbows fit comfortably between your legs at the bottom of the movement.

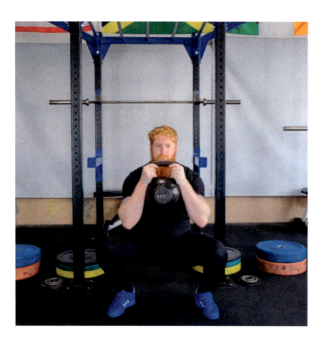

1. Pick up a weight (kettlebell, dumbbell, or plate) and hold it up high at your chest – like you are bringing a large goblet towards your mouth.
2. Take a shoulder-width stance, with your toes pointing to the front or slightly outwards (no more than 30 degrees).
3. Initiate the movement with your hips, driving the glutes back.
4. As your hips hinge, bend your knees (almost simultaneously).
5. Lower under control, keep your knees in line with your toes.
6. Keep your elbows in, so that when you squat down, they comfortably fit in between your legs.
7. Once you have reached the appropriate depth, drive back up out of the squat.
8. Depending on the weight being used, complete 2-3 sets of 10-15 reps.

BACK SQUAT

The back squat is considered by most to be the king of the squats because it allows for the most load to be lifted.

It is the first of three competitive Powerlifts (back squat, bench press, and deadlift) and is usually the foundation of most strength programs.

During the back squat, the barbell is held on your upper back. However, there are two distinct positions on the back that will affect the mechanics of the squat:

- High Bar Position – top of the traps.

- Low Bar Position – 2-3 inches lower than the high bar position (across the spine of the scapula).

There are pros and cons to each position and the various squat styles that are used for each. Therefore, the position you use comes down to your personal preference and your needs and goals – as I usually recommend, incorporate both if you can.

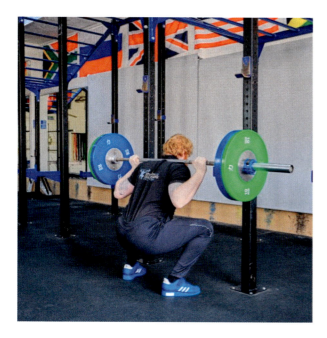

1. Set the barbell on the rack at upper chest height.
2. Grab the barbell 1-2 palms wider than shoulder-width with a comfortable grip (either full or false grip).
3. Move your head under the barbell, placing the barbell into your preferred position on your traps.
4. Walk under the barbell so that your hips are directly underneath it.
5. Lift the barbell up off the rack with your legs and take 2-3 short strides backward.
6. Adopt your squatting stance.
7. Take a big gulp of air, brace your core and use the Valsalva maneuver and pull down on the barbell.
8. Initiate the squat with your hips, driving your glutes back, and bend your knees.
9. Sit back to the point where you break parallel, and your hip crease dips just below the top of your kneecaps, or as deep as you can go while maintaining good form.
10. Drive back up out of the squat.
11. At the top, exhale and get ready for the next rep.
12. Complete 3-5 sets of 1-8 reps.

KNEE VALGUS

Knee valgus involves the knees falling inwards and is a common fault – the opposite of knee valgus is knee varus, which involves the knees pushing outwards.

A common cue is, "push your knees out during the squat," which maximizes the hip abductors / external rotators' engagement and increases tension, increasing performance and preventing knee valgus. However, although this can be a great cue, if an individual is tight through the external rotators (glutes) and weak through the groin and inner thighs, the cue can place excessive stress through the inner thighs and cause the feet to turn outwards as they squat.

Some knee valgus is normal, and it is expected to some degree when lifting maximal loads – elite strength athletes will often experience huge amounts of knee valgus. However, if knee valgus is present at bodyweight or moderate loads, then it shows a clear lack of control, and there are a few simple drills we can use to increase muscle engagement and maintain better control of the legs throughout the squat.

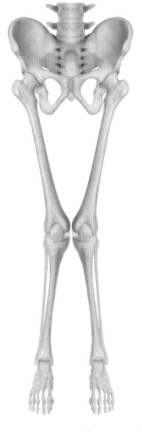 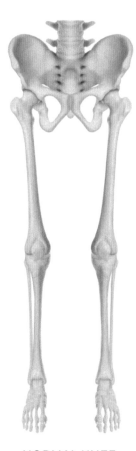 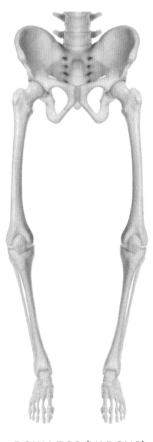

KNOCK KNEE (VALGUS) NORMAL KNEE BOW LEGS (VARGUS)

As mentioned previously, the initial key is the conscious engagement of the correct technique (make the client aware of the issue). From there, we can use Reactive Neuromuscular Techniques (RNT's) to reinforce what needs to be done.

RNT's use resistance bands to pull a joint / limb into the position we DON'T want. Therefore, the muscles that counter this will be forced to work harder.

On top of using RNTs to reinforce muscle engagement and the right technique, several exercises are key to building a muscle that is integral for stability, the gluteus medius.

- Side-lying leg raises.
- Lateral band walks.

Ensuring the gluteus medius is strong is also essential for tensor fasciae latae (TFL) and iliotibial band (ITB) health. If the gluteus medius is not pulling its weight, it can cause the TFL to overwork and the ITB to become sore (a very common problem in runners).

When performing lateral band walks, having a loop band around the feet increases the glute engagement. It also increases the engagement of the intrinsic muscle of the feet and encourages a proper arch.

Flat feet can be a smoke signal for weak glutes. However, genetics also play a major role, and unfortunately, having flat feet can cause the knees to fall inwards when you squat.

Note: An individual might be flat-footed on one side, causing valgus on one side.

To build extra strength in the feet, we can stand on one leg and concentrate on pressing into the floor with the three points of contact – the heel, the big toe, and the little toe.

REACTIVE NEUROMUSCULAR TECHNIQUE:

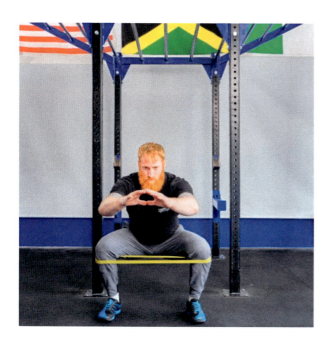

1. Place a small loop band around your knee – this can be above or below your knees.
2. Adopt your squatting stance.
3. Perform squat and as you do so, push your legs against the band – this drill can be performed even with heavy loads on the barbell.
4. Complete 2-3 sets of 5-10 reps.

THE BUTT WINK

The butt wink is a common term used to refer to lumbar flexion (rounding of the lower back) at the bottom of the squat. This happens as the pelvis tucks underneath (posterior pelvic tilt).

A neutral spine is a position that places minimal stress on the structures of the spine. Therefore, when there is a certain degree of lumbar flexion during a squat, there is going to be an increase in stress in the area (especially considering the lumbar vertebrae are flexing and extending under load) – excessive flexion can also result in a loss of tension in the erector muscles and a loss of force transfer.

This is something we should be aware of, especially if there is back pain or a history of lower back issues. However, on the flip side, some degree of lumbar flexion during a deep squat is something we often see in gym-goers and even elite level weightlifters. We know it is not a massive issue for those who can accommodate the stress, but we should consider to what degree it is happening.

During an ass to grass squat, we can expect to see some degree of lumbar flexion in lifters who may not have optimal levers, joint structure, and mobility. However, if we see it happen early on during the eccentric (downward) phase or to an excessive amount, then there are several fixes.

As with most movement faults, the first fix is active engagement. Therefore, bracing the trunk muscles to create more tension around the pelvis will help to maintain its positioning – not only is mind-muscle connection key (consciously engaging muscles), but also mind-body or mind-joint connection (be aware of the positioning of your body).

The best way to build positional strength and awareness is to perform slow repetitions with pauses. Therefore, for the butt wink, performing a slow eccentric goblet squat and pausing at the position where the butt wink occurs can really help us to counter it.

From there, overall squat mobility will help – quads, hip flexor, hamstring, calf, and adductor stretches.

Note: If lumbar flexion is known to exacerbate an individual's back pain, squat depth that results in lumbar flexion should be reduced until a neutral spine can be maintain through a greater ROM.

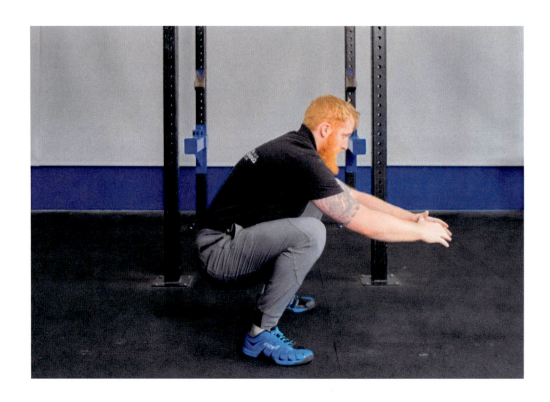

RIBCAGE FLARE

Ribcage flare is where the bottom ribs are raised, meaning the abdominals are lengthened and the lower back has increased extension (hyper-lordosis). This can place greater stress on the lower spine, especially when loads are added to the upper back (a back squat).

Note: Some elite lifters (Powerlifters) may use a technique where they exaggerate the extension of their spine to maximise erector engagement and tension through the posterior chain, helping them to lift heavier loads.

Ribcage flare is something that usually happens because people do not consider rib positioning when setting up for a squat. Therefore, especially when lifting heavier loads, there should be conscious engagement of the abdominals to pull the ribcage down. This both helps to increases intra-abdominal pressure, especially when coupled with the valsalva maneuver, and helps to maintain pelvic positioning throughout the squat.

Just like with the butt wink, this positioning can be practised with slow reps and isometric holds. However, building abdominal strength with anti-extension exercises will also help – this illustrates how "Brace" is fundamental to all movements.

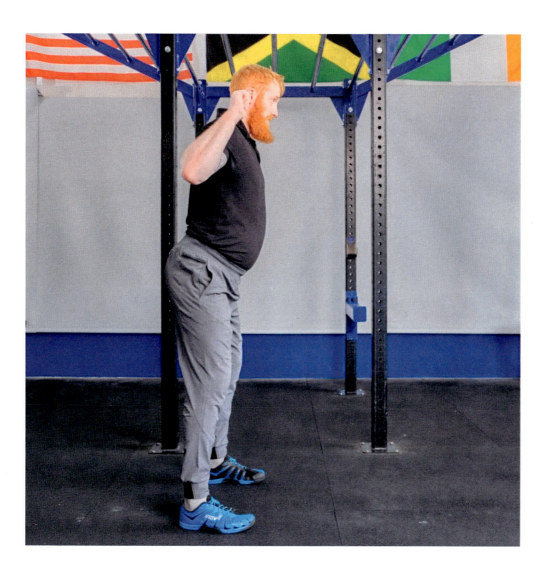

THE HIP SHIFT

The hip shift involves a lifter shifting their weight to one side during the eccentric phase, creating an asymmetrical squat.

This is often due to a strength imbalance where one leg is preferred. For example, a lifter may rely on their right leg. Therefore, as they squat the weight drops to the right side and the left leg can often be seen as slightly raised and abducted to the side.

Step one should therefore be to consciously work the left leg (or whichever leg is not working as hard). Just cueing this can instantly straighten the squat out.

We can test if there is a prominent strength imbalance between the right and left gluteals with a single leg glute bride or hip thrust test. To do this, perform 5-10 reps on each side with 2-3 second holds at the top and see if you notice a prominent difference.

Note: It is common to see a prominent size difference between the right and left gluteal muscles in the bottom of a squat.

If a strength imbalance is identified, this can easily be fixed with extra single leg work.

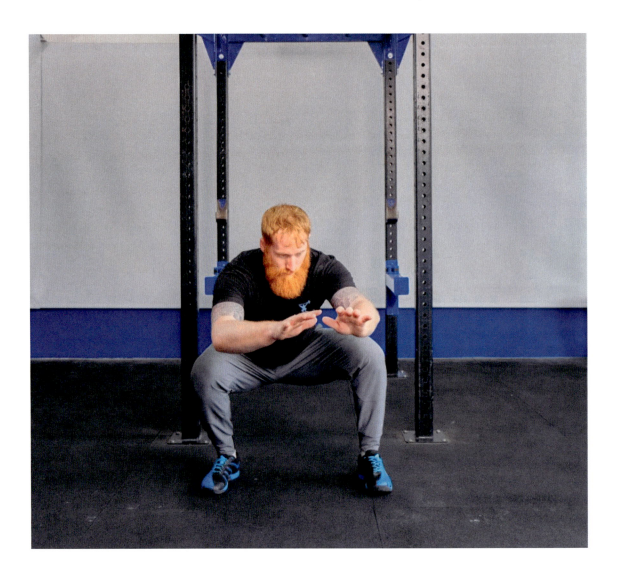

THE GOOD MORNING FAULT

The good morning fault refers to when an individual's knees extend early during the concentric phase of the squat, leaving the muscles of the posterior chain (hamstrings, glutes, and erectors) to finish the work - the name comes from the good morning exercise where you hinge at the hips with a barbell on the upper back.

This is usually down to the quadriceps (which extend the knees) not pulling their weight. The good morning fault can happen during squats, deadlifts, and even single leg movements like step ups – it commonly happens during the deadlift if the lifter tries to take a starting stance that is too deep (it's a deadlift not a squat).

As we come back up past the parallel position, we have often utilised the initial bounce created by the stretch shortening cycle (elasticity of muscles and the stretch reflex) and have got to the position where the pelvis is at its furthest behind the barbell, which is not the most efficient position for the quads.

A great cue is to consciously drive our hips back forward under the barbell, which is a better power position for the quads and can help lifters to power through sticking points. However, it can result in the knees being thrown forward slightly, placing greater stress on them.

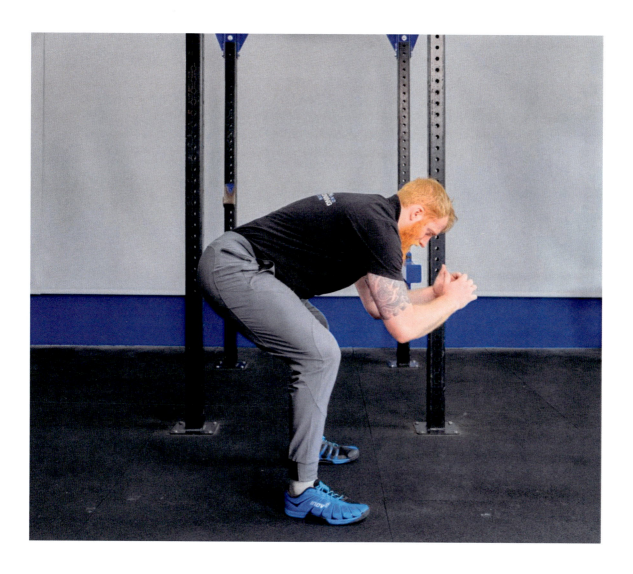

Note: Powerlifters will often use a low bar position (2-3 inches lower on the back), bringing the load closer to the hips and creating a more efficient loading position. From there, they may sit right back with the hips and exaggerate the position with the pelvis behind the barbell, placing the emphasis on the posterior chain – there are clear differences between the way a Powerlifter and Olympic weightlifter may squat.

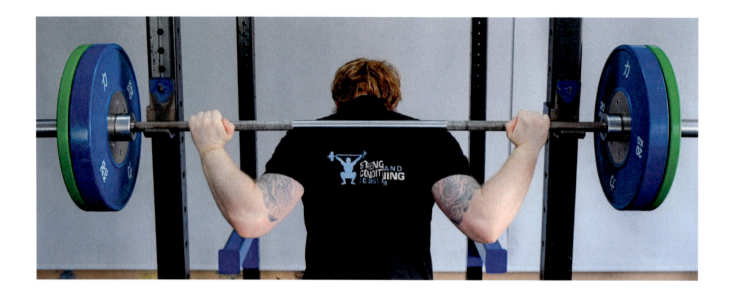

If an individual has an incredibly strong posterior chain, then they can capitalize on this during squats and deadlifts, and their technique may involve less work from the quads with more of a Powerlifting type "squat good morning" style. However, the quads are a huge muscle mass, and we want to get as much out of them as we can.

Squats with the weight loaded to the front (goblet squats, barbell front squats) are going to place more load on the quads and we can use pauses to emphasise this.

We can also add in band exercises to encourage more quad development and engagement:

- **Spanish Squats:** Perform 3-5 sets of 30-60 second holds – you can also perform squats in this position.

- **Terminal Knee Extensions:** Perform 2-3 sets of 15-20 reps on each side.

- **Band Quad Extensions:** Perform 2-3 sets of 10-15 Reps on each side.

Not only will these exercises help to maximise quad engagement, but they will also help to keep the knees in good health by working the quads intensely while placing minimal stress on surrounding structures.

These exercises are a great way to warm-up the quads and knees prior to squatting and can act as maintenance work during times where there is not as much squat volume.

QUADRICEPS DOMINANCE

Quad dominance refers to when the quads are overworking during activities such as running, squatting, lunging, and jumping. This can be down to the quads compensating for a lack of strength in the gluteal and hamstring muscles.

If an individual feels tense through their quads and hip flexors, and a general lack of engagement from their glutes and hamstrings while running and lifting, then it is highly likely that they will benefit from added glute and hamstring work.

This also relates to what is commonly referred to as "glute amnesia" or "glute inhibition". However, we should be very careful that we don't just jump to the conclusion that the gluteal muscles are inhibited, which has become a huge fitness craze in recent years. Often an individual simply hasn't done enough specific hip extension work to build mind-muscle connection and maximise the engagement of these hugely powerful muscle groups during training – it doesn't make sense for the large gluteus maximus muscle to fire maximally when performing small tasks.

Exercises to maximise glute and hamstring engagement:

- Glute bridges and hip thrusts.
- Swiss ball hamstring curls.
- RDLs.

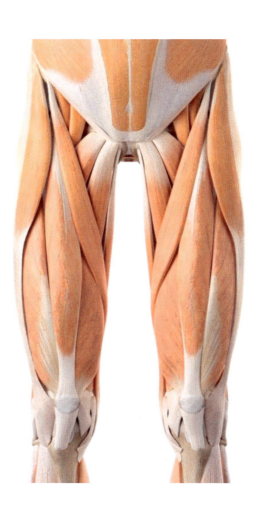

DELOADING THE KNEES

Squats are the foundation of strength development and are brilliant for both structural health and performance. However, there is no doubt that they are stressful on the knee joints and many lifters will experience anterior knee pain at some point, often because of overuse. This is often described at patellofemoral pain syndrome, patella tendinopathy or patella tendinitis. However, it should be diagnosed by an expert.

Remember, all physical training is stress. However, we want adaptive (positive) stress that stimulates adaptations. If we have a sudden spike in frequency and volume (do too much too soon) or intensity (go too hard), it can cause maladaptive (negative) stress which can result in niggles and injuries.

The key is to build strength progressively (progressive overload). However, there is a squat variation that builds huge strength, while minimising the stress on the knees, and that's the **box squat**.

The proper technique for the box squat involves sitting back onto the box so that the shins are vertical at the bottom position. This shin position is referred to as a negative shin angle and results in minimal stress being placed on the knees – the forward tracking of the knees places more stress on the structures (specifically the patella tendon).

Although working with a positive shin angle (ankle dorsiflexed) is integral to athletic performance. The box squat position is more specific to certain members of the population i.e. The elderly – when we get up out of a chair, our shins are vertical and therefore, the box squat couldn't be more specific.

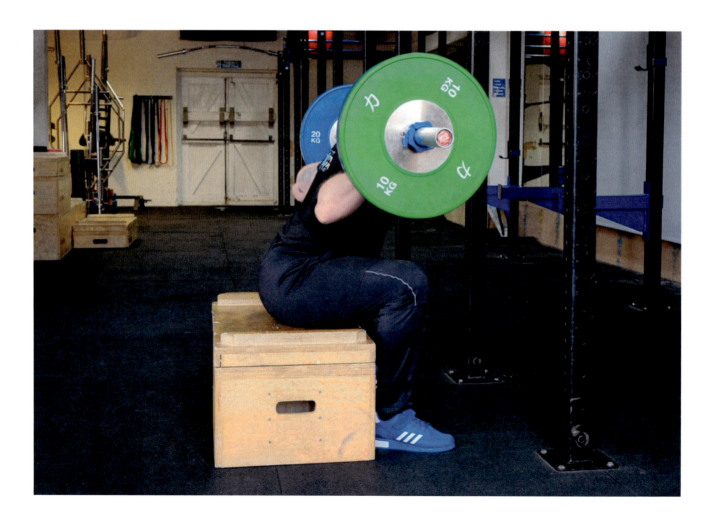

LUNGE

Lunges are just as vital as squats during a warm-up as they too are a fundamental movement pattern.

Any single-leg exercise will be great for warming the legs up and strength development and have the bonus of requiring more stability.

Lunges can be performed forwards, backward, and laterally out to the side, either moving in one direction (walking lunge) or in an alternating fashion where you return to the same starting position each time – striding backward in an alternating fashion is referred to as a reverse lunge.

A forward stride into a lunge is most often used because it is what comes naturally. However, a forward striding lunge can place quite a lot of stress on the front knee. If you have knee pain or find the forward lunge stressful, I recommend using a backward stride (reverse lunge), which unloads a lot of the stress from the front knee.

There are a few foot placement variations that can be used during lunges. I suggest starting from a hip-width stance and lunging forward, leaving a slight gap between each foot (when looking from the front). It's OK to go wider than this if you require extra stability. However, an excessively straddled stance can apply stress to your groin.

WALKING LUNGE:

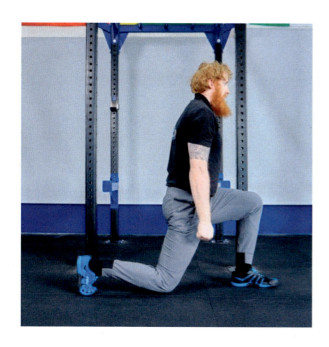

1. Start with a hip-width foot placement.
2. During walking lunges, take a reasonably long stride forward with your right leg. This will allow your left knee to drop comfortably towards the floor while your right knee tracks forward slightly but is still behind your toes.
3. It is fine for your left knee to gently touch the floor. However, this is often avoided to ensure tension remains throughout your body and you don't strike your knee causing bruising - I suggest taking your knee to 1 inch off the floor.
4. As you stride with the front leg and your knee bends, a slight hip hinge will ensure the movement maximises the engagement of not only your quads, but also your hamstrings and glutes. This also ensures your knee doesn't move too far forwards.
5. During walking lunges, you can set the recovering leg down before striding out with it into the next lunge or pass it straight past the supporting leg and into the next lunge.
6. Complete 2-3 sets of 5-10 reps on each side.

LACK OF BALANCE

When it comes to instability and a lack of balance in general, there are two ways we can go about it:

- **General proprioception and balance training:** Single-leg balances etc.

- **Specific movement training:** Regressing the movements and practicing them – drilling the technique.

Proprioception is the sense of knowing where a body part is, and receptors facilitate this in your muscles and tendons called proprioceptors. These receptors detect muscle length changes (muscle spindles) and muscle tension (Golgi tendon organ). For example, when you roll onto the outside of your foot, the muscles on the outer side of your lower leg (peroneal group) detect a change in length. If this lengthening continues, an inversion sprain could occur (damage to the ligaments on the outside of the ankle). Therefore, a signal is sent to the spinal cord, and the spinal cord sends a signal back to involuntarily contract the muscles to prevent injury.

These proprioceptors are constantly sending singles (feedback loops within the nervous system), which helps us maintain optimal positioning. However, proprioception can be impaired when we sustain joint injuries or are prevented from moving for long periods, for example having a leg in a cask for 6 weeks. Therefore, basic proprioception drills should be performed such as standing on one leg – specific equipment like wobble cushions are often used to emphasise the movement at the ankle etc.

Note: Proprioception is an integral component of balance, but balance also requires feedback from the vestibular system (the inner ear) and a degree of muscular strength and endurance, among other factors.

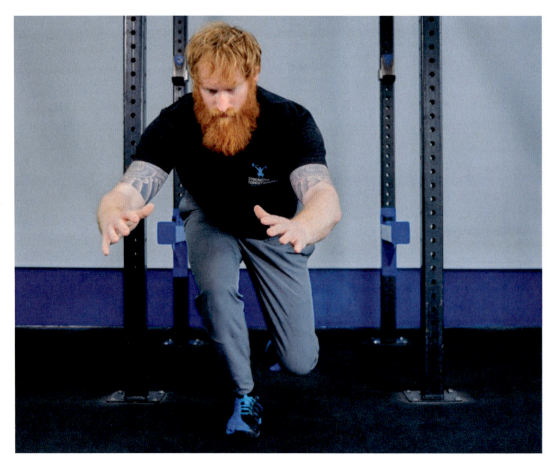

Depending on the ability level and whether someone is recovering from injury, whole sessions may be dedicated to proprioception and balance. However, adding proprioceptive and balance drills into the warm-up or added in at the end of a session is usually sufficient (all movement builds stability to some degree).

We can also increase the work frequency without taking a toll on our lifestyle by using tricks like standing on one leg while doing the dishes or brushing our teeth.

Some of the best proprioceptive and balance drills are:

- Single leg balance variations.

- Single leg swap.

Aside from performing basic proprioceptive and balance drills, the key is specificity. We need to build technique and motor control with the repetition of the exercise to build familiarity.

The easiest way to do this is to regress the movement by providing varying amounts of support:

- Standing between a rack and holding both sides.

- Using a suspension trainer.

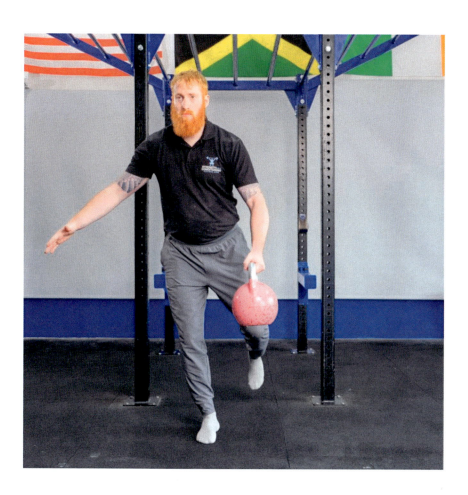

GAIT

Walking and running are basic aspects of human movement and should be something that you do daily. Ironically, they are the most intricate movement patterns to explain in detail.

It's often mistakenly believed that people inherently run with correct form. In reality, muscular imbalances and weaknesses mean that many people have poor running mechanics. This is often compounded by a lack of awareness of the correct form.

Note: You don't have to run with perfect form to run. We are all built differently, and it is normal to have muscular imbalances and a variety of strengths and weaknesses – don't create unnecessary barriers to exercise!

In this section, I will assume that you have no underlying issues and that you also wear suitable footwear (poor footwear is a cause of many problems). This section does not include a gait analysis – instead I will teach you the guidelines for developing optimal form while running.

As individuals, we usually have our own unique, distinctive gait; often it is easy to identify a friend simply by the way they walk and run. When developing your own running technique, it is key to work with your body, not against it. Just because a world class marathon runner runs in a certain way, it doesn't necessarily mean you should mimic their style.

There is, however, professional consensus on "correct" running technique, and you will benefit by observing the best athletes and coaches and adapting your style accordingly. However, if you have run in a particular way all your life, changing your style suddenly can result in structural stresses and injuries. So, take your time and implement changes gradually.

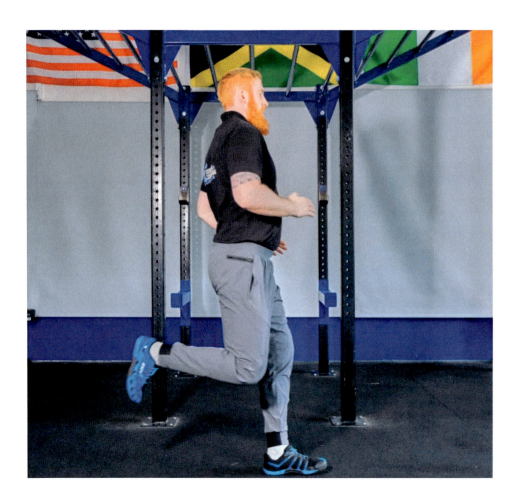

RUNNING MECHANICS

The following guidelines are considered "best practice" when developing a solid running technique (distance running):

Good upper-body posture should be maintained while running, but the torso should tilt forward slightly, driving your weight forward with your chest (sprinters will be more upright).

Your arms should be bent at 90 degrees or less, with your hands in a relaxed fist (choose what suits you). This results in your rear hand coming in line with your hips or slightly higher, and your front arm coming up to your chest. Your arms should swing towards the centre of your body (the midline), but not cross it or punch forward as this can throw you off balance.

As your right leg strides forward, your left arm should swing forward. This not only keeps you balanced, but also creates a diagonal stretch across your front (from right shoulder to left hip), creating elastic energy that when released helps to propel your next stride.

The height at the front and back of the swing will depend on your speed. When sprinting, runners will often bring their front hand up to their face, usually with an open hand (for aerodynamics). However, when covering longer distances, more emphasis is placed on relaxation and balance, rather than forward drive.

Foot strike, which refers to how and where your foot first hits the ground (heel, midfoot or forefoot), is an aspect of running that has become a real bone of contention.

Jump up and down on the spot for a few seconds and you will quickly feel that landing on the midfoot is the most effective way to reduce impact while maximising elastic energy (springiness).

This is a strong argument in favour of midfoot striking. However, top athletes are clearly seen using different styles to great effect – when modifying foot strike, things should be done progressively, as attempting to change your foot strike over a short period of time can lead to injury.

Running should feel natural, so start by working on the bullet points below:

- Maintain good upper body posture with a slight forward tilt of your torso.

- Bend your arms at 90 degrees or less, swinging them forward and back to maintain forward drive and balance – your torso will naturally rotate slightly as you run, but you don't want to overemphasise this by allowing your arms to cross your midline.

- Breathe deeply using your diaphragm and try to regulate your breathing with your strides.

- Land your striding foot directly under your knee.

- Run smoothly and make a conscious effort to strike the floor softly. Push up and off the floor behind you to propel yourself forward. Aim to bring your rear shin to above knee height.

Running form for both sprinters and distance runners is actually quite similar. A sprinter's foot will tend to strike down closer to their centre of mass (under their hips), whereas a distance runner's foot will strike a little further forward. But in both cases, the striding foot should land directly under the knee.

LOADED CARRIES

Loaded carries are some of the most underused exercises. However, there is no doubt that loaded carry variations are some of the best exercises in existence.

Loaded carries strengthen every soft tissue in your body and are also incredibly taxing on your cardio-respiratory system.

If you want to build a strong robust structure, then carries should definitely be programmed in.

The standard carry (farmers carry) involves holding a weight in each hand at your sides, while the suitcase carry, involves holding the weight in one arm only which we saw in the anti-lateral flexion section.

In the videos below, I will show you some of the best carry variants and great grip alternatives to help build strong forearm muscles and robust elbows.

Note: Be cautious not to over program exercise with a huge emphasis on gripping. It is essential to build grip strength progressively. This is because elbow pain can often be caused by overuse.

Carries: Farmers / Suitcase / Front rack / Overhead / Shoulder (Fireman's) / Single shoulder (log) / Baby (Zercher) / Bear hug.

Grip Variations: Full grip / Hook grip / Pincer grip.

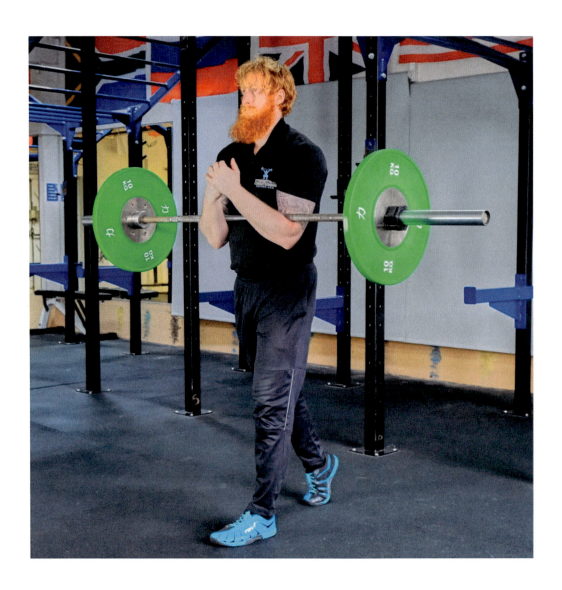

UPPER-BODY COMPOUND MOVEMENTS

Upper body compound movement are split into 2 major categories:

- **Push:** Taking your arms away from your body, working your pectorals, anterior deltoids, and triceps.

- **Pull:** Bringing your arms towards your body, working your back muscles (mid-traps, rhomboids, lats, and posterior deltoids) and biceps.

Both Push and Pull are split down further into 2 categories:

- **Horizontal:** For example, the bench press.

- **Vertical:** For example, the overhead strict press.

Especially when worked with free weights (barbells, dumbbells, and kettlebells), most of the exercises will work the entire body to some extent.

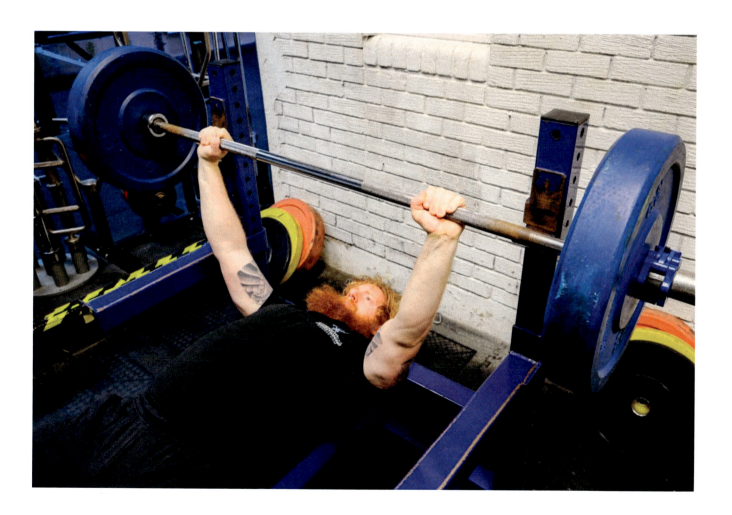

PUSH

Pushing exercises are usually performed horizontally to your front with exercises like the bench press or vertically overhead with exercises like the overhead press. However, you can also press in a downwards fashion with exercises like parallel dips.

The bench press has become the king of pressing exercises, and this is largely due to it being one of the big 3 lifts that Powerlifters compete in (back squat, bench press, and deadlift – in that order). However, the fact many male lifters aspire to have massive pecs (beach body muscle) plays a significant role.

Another reason is that although pushing a heavy barbell on the bench is stressful. It is not as stressful as squatting a heavy barbell, hence why so many leg days are missed.

This being said, although pushing strength is essential for performance, some lifters overdo push exercises, which can result in overuse injuries in the shoulders and elbows specifically.

Note: People will often say the bench press is bad for the shoulders, well, only if you have terrible technique and don't have the strength to accommodate the intensity, volume, and frequency you are doing.

Exercises are rarely "bad." There is just awful exercise prescription, lousy programming of frequency, intensity, volume, and terrible technique.

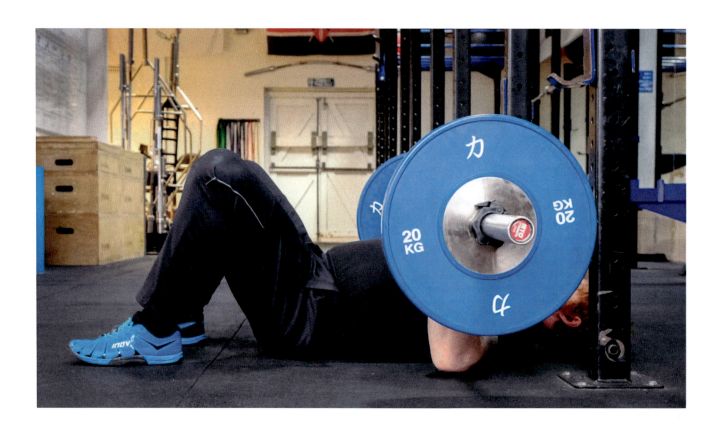

PUSH-UP

Push-ups are a simple exercise in theory, but they are an exercise people often struggle to get right. Not only do you need the chest, shoulder, and triceps strength to push yourself up, you must have the core strength to maintain a rigid trunk.

Common mistakes include allowing the lower back to dip or raising the glutes high in the air. Other errors involve placing the hands too far forward and flaring the elbows out to the side, which places excessive stress on the shoulders.

A common misconception is that you must keep your upper arms locked into your sides while performing push-ups (how people perceive a soldier performing the action). Although this position is fine, some people find it hard to achieve due to their unique anatomy. It's OK for your elbows to be anywhere from directly at your sides to around 45 degrees from your body.

A push-up can be performed while resting on the knees instead of the feet to regress the movement. Kneeling push-ups are fine to use during a fitness class but performing incline push-ups (hands on a raised platform) is a much better way to regress the movement.

Incline push-ups allow you to reduce the strength needed to push yourself up while keeping the movement identical to how it is performed on the floor (with your weight supported between your hands and toes). This setup emphasizes the need for a rigid torso and allows you to lower the incline to increase the effort progressively. Incline push-ups are the best way to progress into performing quality push-ups from the floor.

I often program narrow handed incline push-ups to allow higher reps and create a colossal triceps pump.

Note: A muscle pump refers to the muscle swelling due to the muscle tissue being engorged with blood and the many substances that impact the development of hypertrophy.

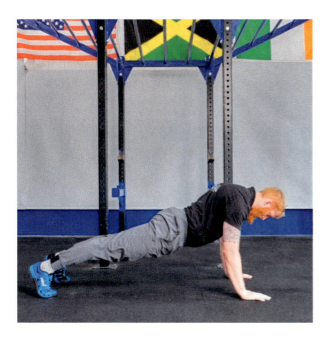

1. Lie chest down on the floor and place your hands under your shoulders.
2. Your feet should be hip width apart.
3. Keep your core braced and drive your palms into the floor, raising yourself up into an extended position.
4. Lower back down under control, until your chest is about 4 inches from the floor, or your chest softly touches the floor.
5. During the push-up, your core should remain braced, and your upper arms should be anywhere from directly at your sides, to 45 degrees from your torso.
6. If performing a push up from your knees, lie flat on the floor, raise your heels off the ground and perform your first rep from there.
7. Complete 2-3 sets of 5-20 reps.

BENCH PRESS

The bench press is by far the most used barbell exercise in a commercial gym environment, with "What can you bench?" seeming to be the only judge of strength.

The bench has gained a reputation for being unfunctional, as you are lying on a bench. However, it is one of the most effective ways of developing your pushing muscles. Therefore, it is incredibly functional.

A great variation of the bench press is the close grip bench press, which emphasizes the triceps. This involves taking a much narrower grip but not to the extent where it negatively affects the wrists – slightly narrower than shoulder-width is usually ideal.

Other variations of the barbell bench press include the decline bench press and the incline bench press.

The decline bench press is performed on a decline bench and dramatically increases the lats' engagement during the press, often allowing heavier loads to be lifted.

The incline bench press is performed on an incline bench (between 35 and 45 degrees) and increases the upper chest and shoulders' engagement. The more you incline the bench, the more shoulder engagement, and less chest engagement there will be.

A common mistake is pulling the barbell off the J-cups with too much force during the incline bench press. This is done during a flat bench press. However, the barbell will often be thrown forward when on an incline bench and end up on the lifter's lap.

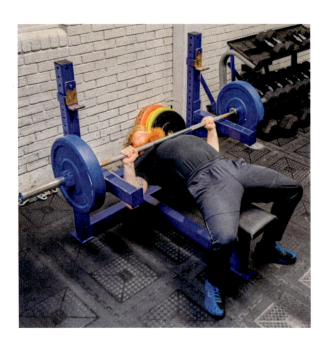

1. Lie on the bench so that your eyes are directly under/slightly behind the barbell.
2. Grab the barbell 1-2 palm's distance wider than shoulder width apart. An ideal grip placement leaves your forearms perpendicular to the barbell at the bottom of the lift.
3. Pull your heels rearwards, push your knees back and drive your soles into the floor.
4. Pull your shoulder blades inwards and down and drive your upper back into the bench. This will facilitate a slight arch in your lower back, leaving two points of contact on the bench (glutes and upper back).
5. Pull the barbell off the J-cups ensuring you do not unset your position.
6. Hold the barbell at the top and take a big gulp of air, brace your core and use the Valsalva manoeuvre.
7. Lower the barbell under control until it comes to your lower chest.
8. Press the barbell up while driving your upper back into the bench.
9. Once you reach the top of the lift, exhale and get ready for the next rep.
10. Complete 3-5 sets of 2-12 reps.

SETTING THE SCAPULA

When pressing horizontally, we set the scapula (shoulder blades), which provides stability, creates tension, increases performance, and keeps the shoulders in good health.

Impingement refers to tissues such as tendons rubbing on another structure, such as a bony prominence like the acromion. It is normal for structures to rub on each other. However, when it becomes excessive, it can cause injury.

The four rotator cuff muscles originate on the scapula. Therefore, when we "set the scapula" during horizontal pressing, we set the scapula in a position that allows us to press weights without overstressing the rotator cuff muscles / tendons.

We must work the muscles that support the shoulder and warm-up the pectoralis and subscapularis before pressing with heavy loads.

- Band Internal & External Rotations / Face Pulls.

- Band Flys.

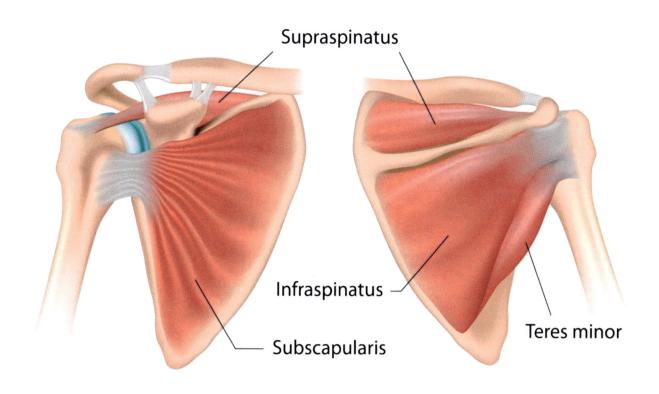

Anterior view   Posterior view

FLARING THE ELBOWS

It is vital to ensure we do not flare our elbows excessively (abduct the shoulder/humerus) while pressing horizontally. Looking at the diagram below the image, if we over abduct the humerus, it will bring the supraspinatus tendon closer to the acromion (bony prominence at the top of the shoulder), increasing the risk of subacromial impingement.

This image illustrates a healthy elbow flare during the bench press.

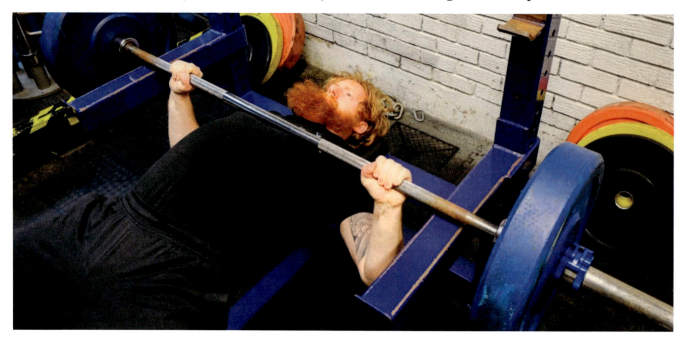

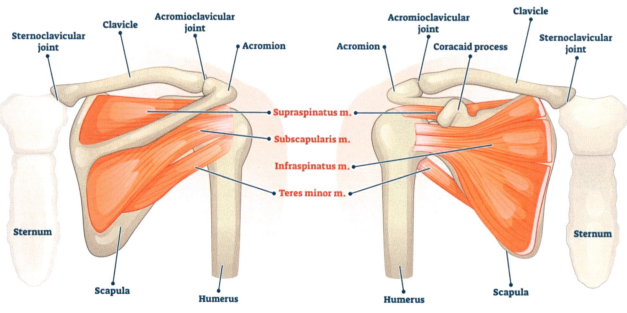

Posterior view   Anterior view

OVERHEAD PRESS

The overhead press (known simply as the press) is by far the most underused barbell exercise. This is because it's not one of the three Powerlifts (squat, bench, deadlift) and is not used in its strict form in Olympic lifting.

It is also one of the most challenging exercises to perform with any reasonable weight compared to the other primary lifts. Hence some people shy away from it.

It takes an unbelievable amount of strength and stability to stand like a pillar and press a heavy weight overhead. Not only that, but it also requires good mobility and lifting mechanics to maintain a press that isn't placing huge amounts of stress on the supporting structures, such as your lower back.

The overhead press places more emphasis on the shoulders and triceps. We don't get as much muscle recruitment from the pectorals, making it is a much harder press than the flat bench press. Not only that, but individuals will also often have insufficient mobility to press overhead, causing compensations. However, this can often be down to poor technique and a lack of engagement of the right scapula mechanics or scapulohumeral rhythm (interaction of the scapula and humerus during movement).

When it comes to pressing overhead, you don't set your scapula. You need your shoulder blades to move throughout the movement to ensure shoulder health.

This movement is often described as a shrugging action. However, you don't want to elevate your shoulders. You want your shoulder blades to rotate upwards. This action is facilitated by the serratus anterior and mid-trapezius.

Upwards rotation involves the upper, inside edge of the scapula (the superior angle) rotating upwards and inwards. A common cue is to imagine the inferior angle (bottom point of the scapula) rotating upwards and outwards towards your armpit – one of the best exercises to practice this is the serratus wall slide.

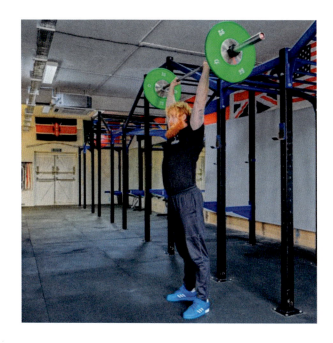

1. Set the barbell on the rack at upper chest height.
2. Grab the barbell slightly wider than shoulder width apart.
3. Bring your elbows forward so they sit directly under the barbell.
4. Stand underneath the barbell and use your legs to lift it off the rack (take it off with your chest). Take 2-3 short strides rearwards and adopt a hip-shoulder width stance.
5. Squeeze your glutes, engage your core and drive your chest upwards and your head back out of the way of the barbell.
6. Take a big gulp of air, brace your core and utilise the Valsalva manoeuvre.
7. Press the barbell upwards without any leg drive (knee bend).
8. Once the barbell passes your head, shrug your upper back. This will bring your torso and head underneath the barbell.
9. Lower the barbell under control.
10. Complete 3-5 sets of 2-12 reps.

OVERHEAD IMMOBILITY

The shoulders have around 165 degrees of flexion from having your hands at your sides. From there, extension through the thoracic spine facilitates the rest to take it to 180 degrees with the arms directly overhead.

If an individual has poor shoulder or thoracic mobility, then the lower back will compensate when you take your arms overhead. This will put excessive stress on the lumbar spine and sacroiliac joints.

Note: Many strength athletes will lean right back during an overhead pressing action, this allows for far more pec engagement and ultimately a stronger press. However, as mentioned previously, the stress levels on the lower back are going to be high.

Shoulder and thoracic mobility exercises:

- Massage ball pec release.

- Pec and anterior delt stretch.

- Band lat stretch.

- Roller thoracic release.

- Shoulder and thoracic mobility stretch.

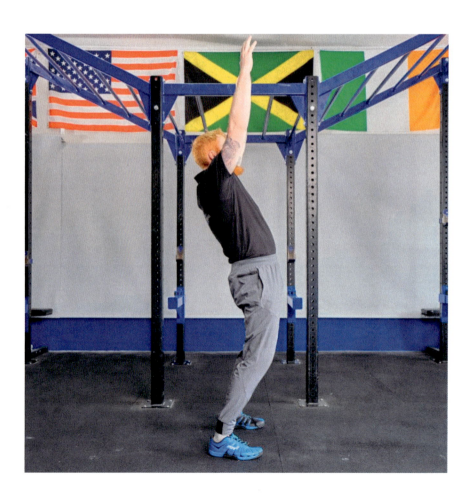

OVERHEAD INSTABILITY

Even with strong pressing muscles, we may still find stability issues while the weight is overhead. Especially while working with the barbell and performing an overhead squat – we will look at the overhead squat in more detail in the last section, "Assessing Movement."

One of the most common faults we see while the arms are loaded overhead, especially while using a wider grip, is one shoulder dropping slightly. This is often a deficit in upper back and external rotator strength on that side.

Fixing a dropping shoulder:

- Band single-arm external rotations and press.

Shoulder stability exercises:

- Overhead holds and carries.

- Hanging band technique (HBT).

- Bottoms up kettlebell press.

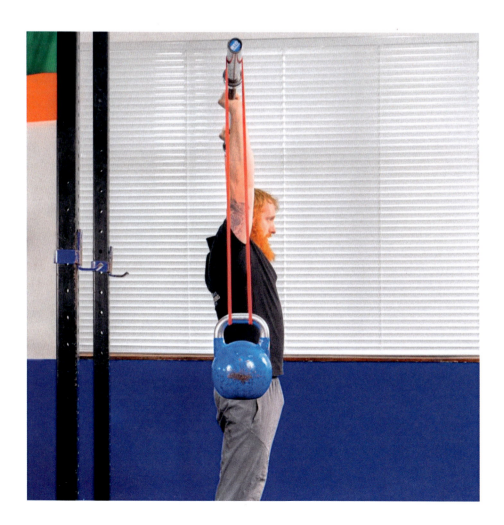

PULL

Although we often describe the deadlift as a pull exercise (pulling the barbell off the floor). This section concentrates on upper body pull exercises.

Pulling exercises are performed horizontally (bent-over rows, single-arm rows) or vertically, either pulling upwards (upright row) or downwards (pull up or lat pull down).

We can perform horizontal pulls on resistance machines such as a seated cable row or with resistance bands attached to a sturdy structure. However, when working with free weights, we adopt a bent-over position to replicate the horizontal pulling action while working against gravity.

Note: When it comes to lifting free weights, we are always working against gravity, which we can imagine as an arrow pointing straight down towards the earth's center. Therefore, the most efficient way to lift a barbell is with a vertical bar path, working directly against gravity's "arrow." However, we can also use an arching motion to increase the mechanical load.

Due to how the body works, most daily activities require us to reach and push forward, creating a bias towards the pushing muscles. Therefore, I recommend incorporating horizontal pulling exercises into your training regime at least 2-3 times a week, even if it is just included in an extended warm-up or cool down after a pressing session.

Horizontal rows are low stress on the shoulder joints but intensely work the upper back, rear deltoids, and rotator cuff, all of which play a role in keeping the joints robust and healthy – I can't overstate the importance of including horizontal pulling exercises into your training.

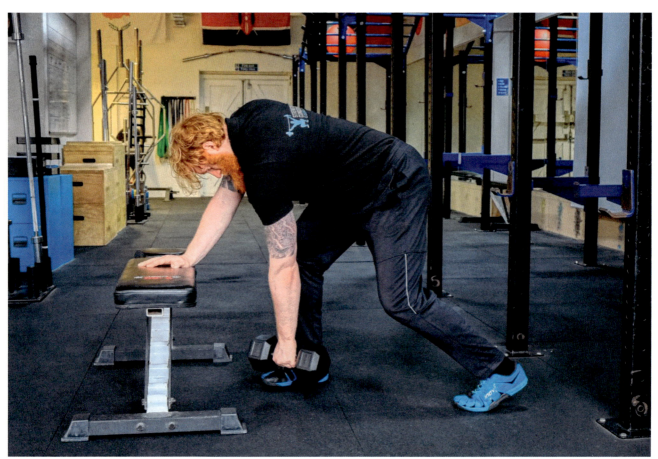

HORIZONTAL PULLING

Upper body pulling exercises develop the back muscles (lats, traps, rhomboids etc), the posterior deltoids and the biceps.

Pulling actions can be performed horizontally, either stood up or sitting and pulling the arms from your front to your sides (usually using resistance bands or a cable machine) or in a bent over position (usually performed with free weights).

If you want healthy shoulders, you want a strong upper back, specifically the muscles that work to stabilise and move the scapula. Many of us also spend much of our day in rounded or slouched postures and as we know, pressing exercises are a favourite of many gym goers. Therefore, it is essential that we include horizontal pulling in our training – pulling frequency can be increased by adding 1 or 2 pulling exercises to the end of a pressing or even lower body session.

When it comes to helping to fix rounded upper back and shoulders, horizontal pulling exercises along with shoulder and thoracic mobility exercises are key:

- Band Horizontal Pulls.

- Band Face Pulls.

- Band Pull Aparts.

Pulling actions can also be performed vertically, either downwards, such as lat pull downs or pull ups (we pull down to pull ourselves up), or upwards with exercises like the upright row.

When we perform horizontal rows from a bent over position, we are getting more engagement from the lats, rhomboids, mid-traps, and posterior deltoids. The more upright we stand from that position, the more the exercise will work the upper traps and medial deltoids.

Pulling upwards (keeping the load close to the body) primarily works the upper traps, whereas pulling downwards, primarily works the lats.

There are several exercises that are ideal for the development of these movements. However, we will look at these after the next slide which discusses elevated and uneven shoulders. This is because there are ways in which we can adapt these exercises to help fix the issues.

- Band lat pull downs.

- Band shrugs.

- Band upright rows.

ELEVATED AND UNEVEN SHOULDERS

One of the most common faults we see is elevated shoulders (on both sides) or uneven shoulders.

People often carry a lot of stress in their upper back, causing them to hunch. It is also common to see people training in hunched postures. This is often due to people trying to create more tension and stability around the shoulders. For example, an individual may hunch while performing biceps curls.

We can stretch these muscles to relieve tension. However, it can also be really beneficial to work the opposing muscles (muscles that retract and bring the scapula down) while encouraging a depressed shoulder position – when we work the opposing muscles, we get reciprocal inhibition (one relaxes to allow the other to contract).

One of the best ways to do this is to perform a downward pulling action from a high anchor point to your front and to really concentrate on keeping the shoulders depressed throughout the movement – ingrain the correct form.

When it comes to the shoulders being uneven, it can quite often be a domino effect, potentially caused by scoliosis or a lateral pelvic tilt. However, a difference between size and muscle tension can be quite prominent between the upper traps and therefore, we can also include unilateral work to build the undeveloped side:

- Band Unilateral Shrugs.
- Band Unilateral Upright Rows.

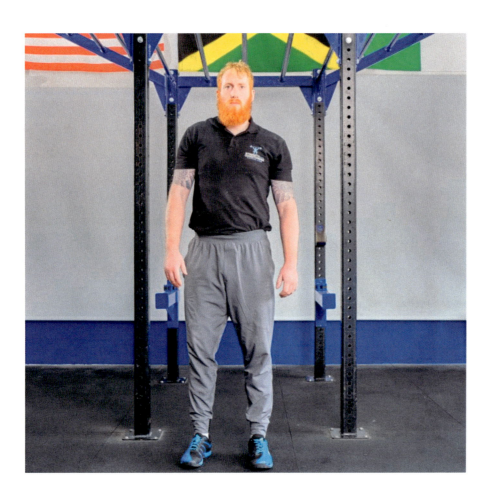

PULL-UP

Pull-ups involve pulling yourself up on a bar with your forearms pronated and your palms facing away from you.

On the other hand, Chin-ups involve the same action, but with the forearms supinated and your palms facing you. Therefore, there is far more biceps engagement, and people tend to feel they can contract their lats harder, making the chin-up easier than the pull-up.

Both variations are brilliant exercises. However, pulling from a pronated grip is generally more specific to real-life and sporting situations like climbing a wall or rock climbing. Therefore, the pull-up is often considered to be the primary variation.

I suggest using both variations and using a neutral grip (palms facing each other), which are often built into various pull-up bar setups or rigs. You can also pull up with an alternate grip on a single bar and take your head to either side of the bar or use a V-bar grip to do the same action.

Pull-ups can be regressed using resistance bands or even supporting your weight with one leg on a box or progressed by adding weight with a dip belt or a dumbbell between your legs.

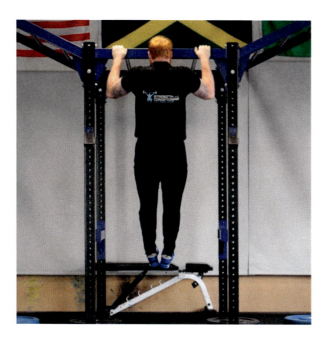

1. Grab the pull-up bar with a supinated grip.
2. As you take your weight, brace your core and push your feet forward slightly to take them off the floor. This position keeps your pelvis in a neutral position (the optimal posture) – having your knees bent with your feet to the rear, slacks your core and can result in your pelvis tilting forward (this can cause lower back pain).
3. Don't be a deadweight, allowing your shoulder joints to distract (joint pulling from its socket). Instead keep your shoulder blades pulled back so the musculature is engaged.
4. Use mind-muscle connection to ensure maximal engagement of your lats and biceps.
5. Pull hard with your back and biceps to bring your chin over, or your chest up to the bar.
6. Lower back down under control, keeping tension in your back at the bottom.
7. Complete 3-5 sets of 2-10 reps – use bands to regress the movement if needed.

BARBELL BENT-OVER ROW

The bent-over row is the primary lift when it comes to upper body pull, often being described as one of the Big 4: Squat, Press, Deadlift, Bent-Over Row.

A pronated grip is often used for barbell rows as this is the grip most used with other barbell exercises. However, a supinated grip will place more emphasis on your biceps, and the EZ bar is often used for comfort on the wrists.

Using a supinated grip pulls your elbows in and, therefore, is a great exercise for building the mid-back and rhomboids. Whereas during a bent-over row with a pronated grip, you will often find you can get more eccentric loading through the latissimus dorsi.

The bent-over row can be performed from any back angle you choose (the back angle is made up between your torso and the floor). The conventional row position is around midway between standing straight up and bending forward with your torso parallel to the floor (45-65 degrees). When performing bent-over rows from a more upright position, it is referred to as a Yates row, named after the bodybuilder and 6 x Mr. Olympia Dorian Yates.

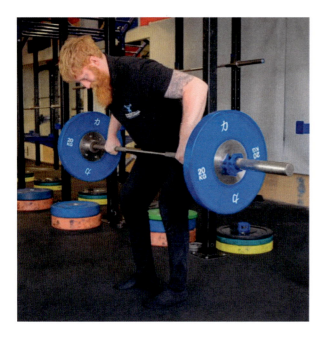

1. Pick the barbell up with a pronated or supinated grip, ensuring you use proper technique to do so (deadlift).
2. Hinge at your hips by pushing your glutes (buttocks) back and allowing your torso to drop forward.
3. As you hinge, bend your knees slightly to bring the barbell to your knees or slightly below (this depends on limb lengths).
4. Adopt the back angle you will be working from. This shouldn't change during the pulls. However, some lifters will use a slight jerking action when working with heavier loads.
5. Pull the barbell up to just above your navel and control it as it lowers back down to the starting position. Allow your shoulders to protract slightly at the bottom to stretch the muscles of your back.
6. Complete 3-5 sets of 5-10 reps.

BARBELL UPRIGHT ROW

Upright rows involve standing upright and pulling a weight from your hips up towards your chin.

A narrow grip is commonly used. However, I prefer to use a slightly wider than shoulder-width (clean grip) or wide snatch grip to perform the lift. This is because a wider grip minimizes the negative stress on the shoulder joints.

When we perform an upright row with a narrow grip, there is considerable shoulder abduction. Some lifters may find this aggravates their shoulders – lifters sometimes complain of an impingement (pinching) feeling at the top of their shoulder(s) (subacromial impingement).

The upright row can be performed with a barbell, EZ bar, or dumbbells, and regardless of what equipment is being used, a great technique tip is to push your chest up high as you perform the upright rows. However, some lifters may lean forward slightly at the bottom of the movement before throwing their torso back during the pull to help them lift more weight.

Throwing your torso back during an upright row is the same as using a jerking action during a bent-over row and is acceptable if you are intentionally trying to lift heavy loads. However, if the aim is to maintain strict form, this should be prevented, and you can enforce this by standing against a wall.

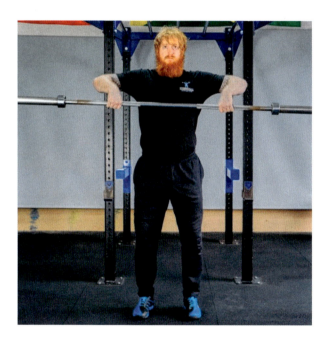

1. Grab the barbell with a clean or snatch grip width.
2. Stand up tall with a proud chest so that the barbell is sitting at or just below the hips.
3. Pull upwards with the arms keeping the barbell close to the body.
4. Pull the elbows upwards and outwards but do not turn the barbell over, bringing the wrists higher than the shoulders.
5. Lower the barbell back down to the hips under control.
6. Perform 3-5 sets of 5-15 reps.

SINGLE-ARM ROW

Single-arm rows are great for both single-arm pulling strength and overall shoulder and upper back health.

Like most rows, the single-arm row can be performed strictly or with a jerking action.

When the single-arm row is performed strictly with no movement in the torso, it acts as a great anti-rotation and anti-flexion exercise because the core muscles work hard to maintain the positioning.

Single-arm rows can be performed in a wide or split stance, with one arm supporting you on a bench. However, you can also place the same side's knee on the bench to provide more support.

There are pros to both variations. Having the extra support from the knee on the bench can allow you to concentrate more on the rowing action and maximize the back and biceps muscles' engagement. While only using the single-arm support requires you to create a stable base with your legs and puts more load onto the core and lower back muscles.

Just like the bent-over row, single-arm rows can be performed from different back angles. The kneeling supported version usually places your torso in a parallel position to the floor with your shoulder level width, or slightly higher than your hips. Whereas the single-arm supported variation usually positions your shoulders much higher than your hips.

The higher your shoulders during a single-arm row, the more the emphasis shifts from your rhomboids to your upper traps.

A famous variation of the single-arm row is the Kroc row, named after an infamous Powerlifter. The Kroc row involves lifting a heavy dumbbell (as heavy as you can) for high reps (20+) in a position where your shoulders are higher than your hips. This variation is unbelievable for building grip strength. However, it can also be performed with straps.

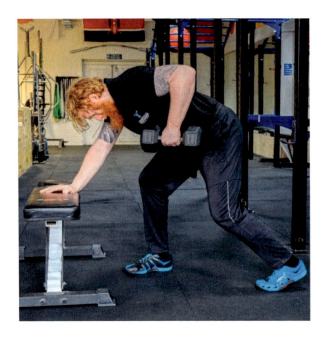

1. Single arm rows can be done with the knee and hand on the same side supported on a bench, or with just one hand on a bench.
2. For the single hand supported row, hinge at your hips and bend your knees slightly, placing your right hand on the bench.
3. Your feet should be slightly wider than shoulder width apart, either side by side or in a split stance.
4. Your torso can be parallel to the floor or angled up.
5. Bend your knees to pick up the dumbbell before raising it up 5-10 inches off the floor.
6. Pull the dumbbell up to your side, ensuring you consciously engage your back and posterior (rear) delts to retract your shoulders.
7. Lower the dumbbell, keeping it under control, and allow your shoulders to protract slightly to stretch the muscles of your back.
8. Complete 2-3 sets of 10-20 reps on each side.

EXAMPLE MOBILITY REGIMES

MORNING STRETCHING ROUTINE

TECHNIQUE	SETS/REPS/TIME	NOTES
Cat-Camel	1x 10 Reps	This routine can be repeated 2-3 times.
Kneeling Lat Stretch (Childs Pose)	1x 20-30 Seconds	
Cobra Stretch	1x 20-30 Seconds	
Downward Dog	1x 20-30 Seconds	
Deep Squat Stretch	1x 20-30 Seconds	
World's Greatest Stretch	1x 3 Rotations (Each Side)	

EVENING STRETCHING ROUTINE

TECHNIQUE	SETS/REPS/TIME	NOTES
Wide Stance Hamstring Stretch	2-3x 20-30 Seconds (Each Side)	
Couch Stretch	1x 1-2 Minutes (Each Side)	
Knees to Chest Stretch	1x 1 Minute (Each Side)	
Lying QL Stretch	1-2x 1 Minute (Each Side)	
Cobra Stretch	1x 1-2 Minutes	
Lying Lat Stretch (Childs Pose)	1x 1-2 Minutes	
Side Lying Thoracic Rotations	1x 5-10 Reps (Each Side)	

TOTAL BODY ROLLING ROUTINE

TECHNIQUE	SETS/REPS/TIME	NOTES
Rolling Feet	1x 20-30 Seconds	Roll both sides of the body at the same time or separately. For total body rolling and stretching, follow each release technique with an applicable stretch.
Rolling Calves	1x 20-30 Seconds	
Rolling Hamstrings	1x 20-30 Seconds	
Rolling Glutes	1x 20-30 Seconds	
Rolling Quads & Outer Thighs	1x 20-30 Seconds	
Rolling Adductors	1x 20-30 Seconds	
Rolling Thoracic Spine	1x 20-30 Seconds	
Rolling Lats	1x 20-30 Seconds	
Rolling Pecs	1x 20-30 Seconds	

TOTAL BODY STRETCHING ROUTINE

TECHNIQUE	SETS/REPS/TIME	NOTES
Heel Drop Calf Stretch	1x 30-60 Seconds (Each Side)	If applicable, bilateral, or unilateral versions of a stretch can be chosen.
Seated (Floor) Hamstring Stretch	1x 30-60 Seconds (Each Side)	
Lying Quad Stretch	1x 30-60 Seconds (Each Side)	
Pigeon Glute Stretch	1x 30-60 Seconds (Each Side)	
Lying QL Stretch	1x 30-60 Seconds (Each Side)	
Cobra Stretch	1x 30-60 Seconds	
Lying Pec Stretch	1x 30-60 Seconds (Each Side)	
Side Lying Thoracic Rotations	1x 30-60 Seconds (Each Side)	
Wall Triceps & Lat Stretch	1x 30-60 Seconds (Each Side)	
Wall Biceps Stretch	1x 30-60 Seconds (Each Side)	
Forearm Flexor & Extensor Stretch	1x 30-60 Seconds (Each Side)	
Trap Stretch	1x 30-60 Seconds (Each Side)	

DESK ROUTINE

Here's a great stretching protocol that you can carry out while at your desk – this can be performed every 40-60 minutes if needed.

TECHNIQUE	SETS/REPS/TIME	NOTES
Seated Thoracic Rotations	1x 20-30 Seconds (Each Side)	This routine can be repeated 2-3 times.
Neck Extensor Stretch	1x 20-30 Seconds	
Seated Trapezius Stretch	1x 20-30 Seconds (Each Side)	
Scalenes & SCM Stretch	1x 20-30 Seconds (Each Side)	

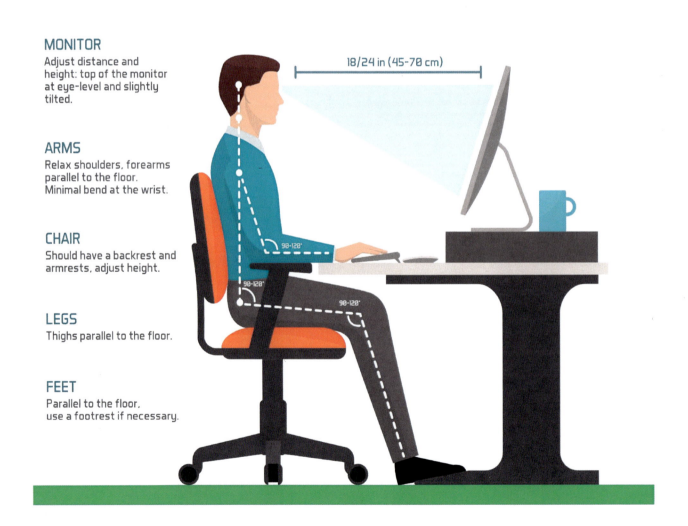

MONITOR
Adjust distance and height: top of the monitor at eye-level and slightly tilted.

ARMS
Relax shoulders, forearms parallel to the floor. Minimal bend at the wrist.

CHAIR
Should have a backrest and armrests, adjust height.

LEGS
Thighs parallel to the floor.

FEET
Parallel to the floor, use a footrest if necessary.

18/24 in (45-70 cm)

HEALTHY HIPS ROUTINE

TECHNIQUE	SETS/REPS/TIME	NOTES
Rolling Glutes	1x 60-90 Seconds (Each Side)	During lying hamstring strap stretch, drop the leg to each side to stretch the inner and outer thighs.
Pigeon Glute Stretch	1x 1-2 Minutes (Each Side)	
Lying Strap Hamstring Stretch	1x 1-2 Minutes (Each Side)	
Frog Stretch	1x 1-2 Minutes	
90/90 Stretch	2-3x 30-60 Seconds (Each Side)	

HEALTHY SHOULDERS ROUTINE

TECHNIQUE	SETS/REPS/TIME	NOTES
Rolling Lats	1x 60-90 Seconds (Each Side)	Slow and controlled rolling.
Wall Lat & Triceps Stretch	1x 1-2 Minutes (Each Side)	
Rolling Pecs	1x 60-90 Seconds (Each Side)	
Wall Pec Stretch	1x 1-2 Minutes (Each Side)	
Anterior Deltoid Stretch	1x 1-2 Minutes (Each Side)	
Medial-Posterior Deltoid Stretch	1x 1-2 Minutes (Each Side)	
Dowel Internal Rotator Stretch	2-3x 30-60 Seconds (Each Side)	
Dowel External Rotator Stretch	2-3x 30-60 Seconds (Each Side)	

POST RUN ROUTINE

TECHNIQUE	SETS/REPS/TIME	NOTES
Rolling Calves	1x 60-90 Seconds (Each Side)	Slow and controlled rolling.
Hell Drop Calf Stretch	2x 1-2 Minutes (Each Side)	If the routine is used pre-run, reduce the times to sub 30 seconds for both the rolling and stretching (pick drills that are relevant).
Rolling Peroneus/Tibialis Anterior	1x 60-90 Seconds (Each Side)	
Seated Top of Foot Stretch	1x 30-60 Seconds	Perform calf stretches with straight and bent knees for gastrocnemius and soleus.
Rolling Hamstrings	1x 60-90 Seconds (Each Side)	
Hurdler Hamstring Stretch	1x 1-2 Minutes (Each Side)	
Rolling Quads	1x 60-90 Seconds (Each Side)	
Couch Stretch	1x 1-2 Minutes (Each Side)	
Rolling Glutes	1x 60-90 Seconds (Each Side)	
Figure Four Glute Stretch	1x 1-2 Minutes (Each Side)	

POST SQUAT / LOWER BODY ROUTINE

TECHNIQUE	SETS/REPS/TIME	NOTES
Rolling Quads	1x 60-90 Seconds (Each Side)	Slow and controlled rolling.
Lying Quad Stretch	1x 1-2 Minutes (Each Side)	
Rolling Glutes	1x 60-90 Seconds (Each Side)	
Figure Four Glute Stretch	1x 1-2 Minutes (Each Side)	
Rolling Hamstrings	1x 60-90 Seconds (Each Side)	
Hurdler Hamstring Stretch	1x 1-2 Minutes (Each Side)	
Butterfly Stretch	1x 1-2 Minutes	
Rolling Calves	1x 60-90 Seconds (Each Side)	
Standing Calf Stretch	1x 1-2 Minutes (Each Side)	

POST DEADLIFT ROUTINE

TECHNIQUE	SETS/REPS/TIME	NOTES
Knees to Chest Stretch	1x 1-2 Minutes (Each Side)	Slow and controlled rolling.
Iron Cross Stretch	1x 1-2 Minutes (Dynamic)	
Cobra Stretch	1x 30-60 Seconds	
Thoracic Extension Drill	1x 60-90 Seconds	
Side Lying Thoracic Rotations	1x 5-10 Reps (Each Side)	
Rolling Glutes	1x 60-90 Seconds (Each Side)	
Figure Four Glute Stretch	1x 1-2 Minutes (Each Side)	
Rolling Hamstrings	1x 60-90 Seconds (Each Side)	
Standing Hamstring Stretch	1x 1-2 Minutes (Each Side)	
Rolling Quads	1x 60-90 Seconds (Each Side)	
Standing Quad Stretch	1x 1-2 Minutes (Each Side)	

POST UPPER PUSH ROUTINE

TECHNIQUE	SETS/REPS/TIME	NOTES
Dowel Internal Rotator Stretch	1x 1-2 Minutes (Each Side)	Slow and controlled rolling.
Dowel External Rotator Stretch	1x 1-2 Minutes (Each Side)	
Rolling Pecs	1x 60-90 Seconds (Each Side)	
Band Pec Stretch	1x 1-2 Minutes	
Anterior Deltoid Stretch	1x 1-2 Minutes (Each Side)	
Medial-Posterior Deltoid Stretch	1x 1-2 Minutes (Each Side)	
Barbell Rolling Triceps	1x 60-90 Seconds (Each Side)	
Standing Triceps Stretch	1x 1-2 Minutes (Each Side)	

POST UPPER PULL ROUTINE

TECHNIQUE	SETS/REPS/TIME	NOTES
Lying Knee Rolls	1x 1-2 Minutes (Dynamic)	Slow and controlled rolling.
Barbell Rolling Lats	1x 60-90 Seconds (Each Side)	
Standing Lat Stretch	1x 1-2 Minutes (Each Side)	
Rhomboids Stretch	1x 1-2 Minutes	
Standing Trap Stretch	1x 30-60 Seconds (Each Side)	
Quadruped Thoracic Rotations	1x 5-10 Reps (Each Side)	
Lying Barbell Rolling Biceps	1x 60-90 Seconds (Each Side)	
Biceps Wall Stretch	1x 1-2 Minutes (Each Side)	

PRE-OLYMPIC WEIGHTLIFTING ROUTINE

TECHNIQUE	SETS/REPS/TIME	NOTES
Rolling Feet	1x 30-60 Seconds (Each Side)	Roll at a good tempo that will encourage circulation and help to raise deep muscle temperature.
Rolling Calves	1x 30-60 Seconds (Each Side)	
Heel Drop Calf Stretch	1x 30-60 Seconds (Each Side)	
Rolling Hamstrings	1x 30-60 Seconds (Each Side)	
Rolling Glutes	1x 30-60 Seconds (Each Side)	
Rolling Quads & Outer Thighs	1x 30-60 Seconds (Each Side)	
Rolling Pecs	1x 30-60 Seconds (Each Side)	
Rolling Lats	1x 30-60 Seconds (Each Side)	
Band Lat Stretch	1x 30-60 Seconds (Each Side)	
Rolling Thoracic Spine	1x 30-60 Seconds (Each Side)	
Thoracic Extension Drill	1x 30-60 Seconds (Each Side)	

EXAMPLE STRENGTH REGIMES

Most of the workouts in this section can be completed 1-3 times a week. Individual exercises can be performed with successive sets, or a circuit can be performed (perform each exercise back-to-back and repeat 2-3 times – take 30-60 seconds rest between rounds of the circuit).

BODYWEIGHT BASICS

EXERCISE	SETS/REPS/TIME	REST
Bodyweight Hip Hinge	3x10	15-30 Seconds
Bodyweight Squat	3x10	15-30 Seconds
Bodyweight Reverse Lunge	3x5 (Each Side)	15-30 Seconds
Push-Up	3x10	15-30 Seconds
Pull-Up (Band Assisted if Needed)	3x5	15-30 Seconds

STRONG AND HEALTHY SHOULDERS

EXERCISE	SETS/REPS/TIME	REST
Serratus Wall Slides	3x5	15-30 Seconds
Single-Arm Band Fly	3x15	15-30 Seconds
Band Pull Apart	3x15	15-30 Seconds
Band Face Pull	3x15	15-30 Seconds
YWT	3x5 Cycles	15-30 Seconds
Straight-Arm Lat Pulldown	3x10	15-30 Seconds

STRONG & HEALTHY ELBOWS & WRISTS

EXERCISE	SETS/REPS/TIME	REST
Zottman Curl	3x8	30-60 Seconds
Triceps Pushdown	3x15	30-60 Seconds
Wrist Curl (Flexion – Palms Up)	3x10	30-60 Seconds
Wrist Curl (Extension – Palms Down)	3x10	30-60 Seconds

STRONG & HEALTHY HIPS

EXERCISE	SETS/REPS/TIME	REST
Glute Bridge	3x20	15-30 Seconds
Lateral Band Walk	3x20 Strides (Each Side)	15-30 Seconds
Standing Psoas March	3x10 (Each Side)	15-30 Seconds
Band Good Morning	3x10	15-30 Seconds
Fire Hydrant	3x10 (Each Side)	15-30 Seconds

STRONG & HEALTHY KNEES

EXERCISE	SETS/REPS/TIME	REST
Band Glute Bridge	3x20	15-20 Seconds
Lateral Band Walk	3x20 (Each Side)	15-20 Seconds
Standing Psoas March	3x10 (Each Side)	15-20 Seconds
Terminal Knee Extension	3x15 (Each Side)	5-10 Seconds
Spanish Squat	4x40 Seconds	30-60 Seconds

STRONG & HEALTHY ANKLES

EXERCISE	SETS/REPS/TIME	REST
Heel Drop Calf Raise	4x15	1 Minute
Seated Soleus Raise	4x15	1 Minute
Band Dorsiflexion	4x15	1 Minute
Band Eversion/Inversion	3x10 (Each Side)	30-60 Seconds
Lateral Band Walk	3x20 Strides (Each Side)	15-30 Seconds

STRONG & HEALTHY LOWER BACK

EXERCISE	SETS/REPS/TIME	REST
Bird Dog	3x5 (Each Side)	15-30 Seconds
Donkey Kick Back	3x10 (Each Side)	15-30 Seconds
Band Good Morning	3x10	15-30 Seconds
Dead Bug	3x5 (Each Side)	15-30 Seconds
Pallof Press	3x5 (Each Side)	15-30 Seconds
Side Plank	2x30 Seconds (Each Side)	15-30 Seconds

CORE DEVELOPMENT

EXERCISE	SETS/REPS/TIME	REST
Sit-Up	3x15	15-30 Seconds
Front Plank	3x30 Seconds	15-30 Seconds
Bird Dog	3x5 (Each Side)	15-30 Seconds
Side Plank	2x30 Seconds (Each Side)	15-30 Seconds
Pallof Press	3x5 (Each Side)	15-30 Seconds

The following workouts are centred around the barbell. We can use percentages of a 1 rep max (most we can lift for 1 repetition) to quantify workloads. However, the training programs below us the RPE Scale is simple and effective.

The RPE (Rating of Perceived Exertion) Scale is a 1-10:

RPE	INTENSITY
1-2	Very easy
3	Easy
4	Moderate
5-6	Somewhat hard
7-8	Hard
9	Very Hard
10	Maximal

LOWER BODY

EXERCISE	SETS/REPS/TIME	REST
Bodyweight Squat	2x10	15-20 Seconds
Goblet Squat	2x10 at RPE 7	20-30 Seconds
Back Squat	5x5 at RPE 9	2-3 Minutes
RDL	4x8 at RPE 8	1-2 Minutes
Walking Lunge	3x6 (Each Side) at RPE 8	1-2 Minutes

DEADLIFT & UPPER PULL

EXERCISE	SETS/REPS/TIME	REST
Deadlift	5x5 at RPE 9	2-3 Minutes
Bent-Over Row	4x10 at RPE 9	1-2 Minutes
Upright Row	4x10 at RPE 8	1-2 Minutes
Single-Arm Row	3x10 (Each Side) at RPE 8	1-2 Minutes
Full Curls	3x10 at RPE 8	1 Minute

UPPER PUSH & PULL

EXERCISE	SETS/REPS/TIME	REST
Bench Press	4x8 at RPE 9	1-2 Minutes
Bent-Over Row	4x8 at RPE 9	1-2 Minutes
Overhead Press	4x8 at RPE 9	1-2 Minutes
Single-Arm Row	3x8 (Each Side) at RPE 9	1-2 Minutes
Triceps Extensions	3x10 at RPE 8	1 Minute
Full Curls	3x10 at RPE 8	1 Minute

UPPER PUSH

EXERCISE	SETS/REPS/TIME	REST
Bench Press	5x5 at RPE 9	2-3 Minutes
Overhead Press	4x10 at RPE 9	1-2 Minutes
Fly	4x8 at RPE 8	1-2 Minutes
Triceps Extensions	3x10 at RPE 8	1 Minute

UPPER PULL

EXERCISE	SETS/REPS/TIME	REST
Pull Up	3x5	1-2 Minutes
Bent-Over Row	4x10 at RPE 9	1-2 Minutes
Upright Row	4x10 at RPE 8	1-2 Minutes
Single-Arm Row	3x10 (Each Side) at RPE 8	1-2 Minutes
Crossbody Hammer Curl	3x6 (Each Side) @RPE 8	1 Minute

SQUAT, PUSH, PULL: 3-WEEK CYCLE

WEEK	EXERCISE	SETS/REPS/TIME	REST
Week 1	Back Squat	4x8 at RPE 8	1-2 Minutes
	Bench Press	4x8 at RPE 8	1-2 Minutes
	Deadlift	3x5 at RPE 8	2-3 Minutes
	Bent-Over Row	3x10 at RPE 8	1-2 Minutes
Week 2	Back Squat	4x5 at RPE 9	2-3 Minutes
	Bench Press	4x5 at RPE 9	2-3 Minutes
	Deadlift	3x3 at RPE 9	2-3 Minutes
	Bent-Over Row	3x8 at RPE 9	1-2 Minutes
Week 3	Back Squat	4x3 at RPE 10	2-3 Minutes
	Bench Press	4x3 at RPE 10	2-3 Minutes
	Deadlift	3x2 at RPE 10	2-3 Minutes
	Bent-Over Row	3x6 at RPE 10	1-2 Minutes

CONCLUSION

This manual has been built from several resources (online courses and eBooks) that I have produced over the years to help my clients, athletes, and students.

Courses & eBooks Featured in this book:

- Muscles & Movement Course.

- Corrective Exercise Course.

- The Movement Muscle Manual V2 eBook.

- Mobility & Flexibility eBook.

The courses include full video tutorials for all the exercises.

I hope you enjoy this manual as much as I enjoyed putting the content together, and I hope it is a useful resource for you for years to come.

Always remember, being an expert is an ongoing project.

Coach Curtis

Become the Expert!

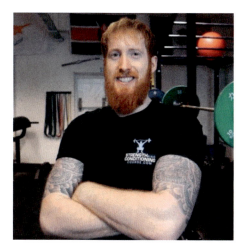

FREE CONTENT

Link and QR Code on the last page.

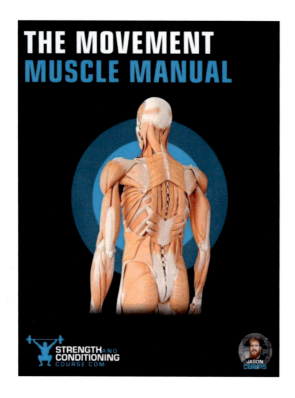

This unique muscle manual categorizes muscles by their movements, giving you a much better understanding of how muscles assist and oppose each other to perform actions.

You also get a FREE second version of the muscle manual, which lists:

- Origin.
- Insertion.
- Action.
- Antagonist.
- Innervation.
- Blood Supply.
- Daily Use.
- Gym Use.

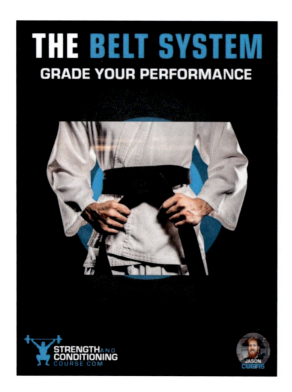

The Belt System was designed as a FUN way for clients and athletes to set targets. However, we were amazed at how popular it became - the increases in motivation have been huge!

There are 5 disciplines, 8 tests per discipline, and 8 coloured belts up for grabs!

- Bodyweight Muscular Endurance.
- Barbell Strength.
- Olympic Weightlifting.
- Speed & Power.
- Endurance.

What belts can you achieve?

OUR COURSES

Link and QR Code on the last page.

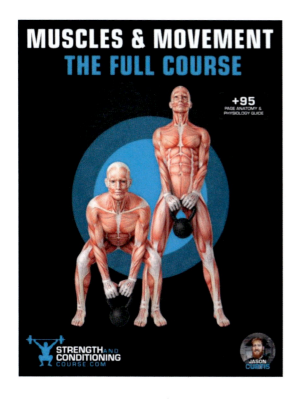

If you want to be an expert, you need an in-depth understanding of functional anatomy - the way muscles facilitate movement and how this relates to training.

In this course, Coach Curtis discusses the intricacies of each slide from his unique muscle manual and has included hours of video tutorials demonstrating how to target each area.

Become a Muscles & Movement Specialist (MMS).

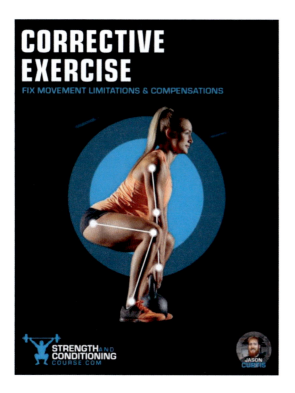

This course is designed for fitness professionals and enthusiasts who want to gain an in-depth understanding of how to fix technique faults and compensation patterns caused by mobility restrictions, muscular imbalances, and asymmetries.

In this course, we look at how to teach fundamental human movements and exercises and explain how to fix over 30 common faults.

Maximize performance and minimize your risk of injury!

Become a Corrective Exercise Specialist (CES).

OUR COURSES

Link and QR Code on the last page.

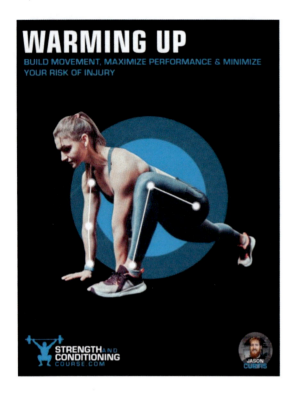

A good session starts with a great warm-up, and there are countless ways to maximize the effectiveness of this essential part of a session.

In this course, we delve deeper into how we can optimize the warm-up protocol to minimize our risk of injury and maximize performance on the subsequent session. We also look at how we create a warm-up that acts as an important part of the session where various physical attributes can be developed long-term.

- Running Drills.
- DROME's.
- Potentiation.

Become a Warming Up Specialist (WUS).

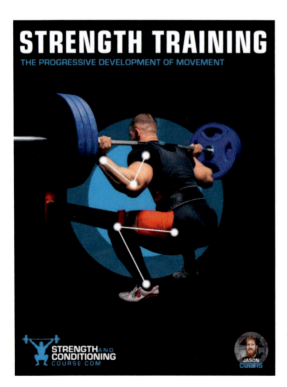

The development of strength is the foundation of physical performance because, before all else, you need the strength in your structures to support the fundamental movements that you carry out each day.

This HUGE course consists of 240+ narrated slides and 4+ hours of video tutorials for over 100 exercises.

Become a Strength Training Specialist (STS).

OUR OTHER BOOKS

Link and QR Code on the last page.

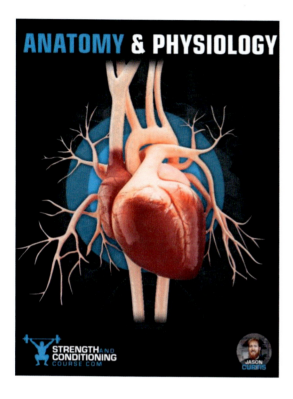

This manual is perfect for those looking to qualify as fitness professionals, experienced coaches looking for a refresh, and enthusiasts looking to learn more about the human body - we make anatomy accessible!

This manual takes a simplified, straight-to-the-point look at nine key sections, with dozens of large, full-colour diagrams and illustrations.

- The Cardiorespiratory System.
- The Skeletal System.
- The Muscular System.
- The Nervous System.
- The Endocrine System.
- The Energy Systems.
- The Digestive System.
- The Components of Fitness.
- Injuries.

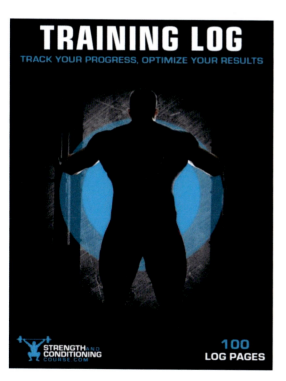

The SCC Training Log has been designed by expert Strength and Conditioning coaches who have years of experience working with athletes and the general public.

What you get within the log:

- How to Quantify Training Loads.
- How to Test.
- Methods of Strength Development.
- How to Program.
- Goals, Strength and Weaknesses and Injury Trackers.
- 1RM Table.
- 100 Log Pages.

All within a convenient A5 logbook.

Check out all our content by using the link below or scanning the QR code:

https://courses.strengthandconditioningcourse.com

BIBLIOGRAPHY

1. American Academy of Orthopaedic Surgeons. (1983). Joint Motion: Method of Measuring and Recording. Chicago: AAOS.

2. Baechle, T., and Earle, R. (2008). Essentials of Strength Training and Conditioning. 3rd edition. Champaign, IL: Human Kinetics.

3. Balady, G.J. et al. (2000). General Principles of Exercise Prescription. In ACSM's Guidelines for Exercise Testing and Prescription. (Franklin, B.A. et al, eds) pp.138. Lippincott Williams and Wilkins.

4. Cheung, K. et al. (2003). Delayed Onset Muscle Soreness: Treatment Strategies and Performance Factors. Sports Medicine, 33(2), pp.145-164.

5. Cook, G. (2011). Movement: Functional Movement Systems: Screening, Assessment, Corrective Strategies. West Sussex: Lotus Pub.

6. Corrigan, B., and Maitland, G.D. (1994), Musculoskeletal and Sports Injuries. Philadelphia, PA: Elsevier Health Sciences.

7. Costanzo, L.S. (2010). Physiology. 4th edition. Philadelphia, PA: Saunders Elsevier.

8. Earle, R.W. and Baechle, T.R. (2004). NSCA's Essentials of Personal Training. Champaign, IL: Human Kinetics.

9. Enoka, R. (1988). Neuromuscular Basis of Kinesiology. Champaign, IL: Human Kinetics.

10. Fleck, S.J. and Kraemer, W.J. (2014). Designing Resistance Training Programs. 4th edition. Champaign, IL: Human Kinetics.

11. Gray, H. (1980. Gray's Anatomy. 36th Edition. Edinburgh: Churchill Livingstone.

12. Kenney, W.L. et al. (2012). Physiology of Sport and Exercise. 5th edition. Champaign, IL: Human Kinetics.

13. McGill, S. (2002). Low Back Disorders: Evidence-Based Prevention and Rehabilitation. Human Kinetics.

14. McGinnis, P.M, (2013). Biomechanics of Sport and Exercise. 3rd edition. Champaign, IL: Human Kinetics.

15. McKinley, M.P. et al. (2012). Human Anatomy. 4th edition. New York: McGraw Hill Education.

16. Muscolino, J.E. (2010). Kinesiology: The Skeletal System and Muscle Function. 2nd edition, Missouri: Mosby.

17. Noakes, T. (2002). The Lore of Running. Champaign, IL: Human Kinetics.

18. Richards, J. (2008). Biomechanics in Clinic and Research. Philadelphia: Churchill Livingstone, Elsevier.

19. Solomon, E.P., Schmidt, R.R. and Adragna, P.J. (1990). Human Anatomy and Physiology. 2nd edition. Florida, USA: Saunders College Publishing.

20. Tortora, G.J. and Derrickson, B.H. (2009). Principles of Anatomy & Physiology. 12th edition. New Jersey: John Wiley & Sons.

21. Waugh, A. and Grant, A, (2014). Anatomy and Physiology in Health and Illness. 11th edition. Philadelphia: Churchill Livingstone, Elsevier.

22. Wilmore, J. and Costill, D. (1999). Physiology of Sport and Exercise. Champaign, IL: Human Kinetics.

23. Zatsiorsky, V.M. (1995). Science and Practise of Strength Training. Champaign, IL: Human Kinetics.

Made in United States
Orlando, FL
08 October 2023

37691255R00168